T0155885

Communications
in Computer and Information Science 1772

Rationale

The CCIS series is devoted to the publication of proceedings of computer science conferences. Its aim is to efficiently disseminate original research results in informatics in printed and electronic form. While the focus is on publication of peer-reviewed full papers presenting mature work, inclusion of reviewed short papers reporting on work in progress is welcome, too. Besides globally relevant meetings with internationally representative program committees guaranteeing a strict peer-reviewing and paper selection process, conferences run by societies or of high regional or national relevance are also considered for publication.

Topics

The topical scope of CCIS spans the entire spectrum of informatics ranging from foundational topics in the theory of computing to information and communications science and technology and a broad variety of interdisciplinary application fields.

Information for Volume Editors and Authors

Publication in CCIS is free of charge. No royalties are paid, however, we offer registered conference participants temporary free access to the online version of the conference proceedings on SpringerLink (http://link.springer.com) by means of an http referrer from the conference website and/or a number of complimentary printed copies, as specified in the official acceptance email of the event.

CCIS proceedings can be published in time for distribution at conferences or as post-proceedings, and delivered in the form of printed books and/or electronically as USBs and/or e-content licenses for accessing proceedings at SpringerLink. Furthermore, CCIS proceedings are included in the CCIS electronic book series hosted in the SpringerLink digital library at http://link.springer.com/bookseries/7899. Conferences publishing in CCIS are allowed to use Online Conference Service (OCS) for managing the whole proceedings lifecycle (from submission and reviewing to preparing for publication) free of charge.

Publication process

The language of publication is exclusively English. Authors publishing in CCIS have to sign the Springer CCIS copyright transfer form, however, they are free to use their material published in CCIS for substantially changed, more elaborate subsequent publications elsewhere. For the preparation of the camera-ready papers/files, authors have to strictly adhere to the Springer CCIS Authors' Instructions and are strongly encouraged to use the CCIS LaTeX style files or templates.

Abstracting/Indexing

CCIS is abstracted/indexed in DBLP, Google Scholar, EI-Compendex, Mathematical Reviews, SCImago, Scopus. CCIS volumes are also submitted for the inclusion in ISI Proceedings.

How to start

To start the evaluation of your proposal for inclusion in the CCIS series, please send an e-mail to ccis@springer.com.

Buzhou Tang · Qingcai Chen · Hongfei Lin ·
Fei Wu · Lei Liu · Tianyong Hao ·
Yanshan Wang · Haitian Wang
Editors

Health Information Processing

8th China Conference, CHIP 2022
Hangzhou, China, October 21–23, 2022
Revised Selected Papers

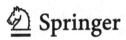 Springer

Editors
Buzhou Tang ⓘ
Harbin Institute of Technology, Shenzhen
Shenzhen, China

Hongfei Lin ⓘ
Dalian University of Technology
Dalian, China

Lei Liu
Fudan University
Shanghai, China

Yanshan Wang
University of Pittsburgh
Pittsburgh, USA

Qingcai Chen ⓘ
Harbin Institute of Technology, Shenzhen
Shenzhen, China

Fei Wu
Zhejiang University
Hangzhou, Zhejiang, China

Tianyong Hao ⓘ
South China Normal University
Guangzhou, China

Haitian Wang ⓘ
The Chinese University of Hong Kong
Hong Kong, China

ISSN 1865-0929   ISSN 1865-0937 (electronic)
Communications in Computer and Information Science
ISBN 978-981-19-9864-5   ISBN 978-981-19-9865-2 (eBook)
https://doi.org/10.1007/978-981-19-9865-2

This Springer imprint is published by the registered company Springer Nature Singapore Pte Ltd.
The registered company address is: 152 Beach Road, #21-01/04 Gateway East, Singapore 189721, Singapore

Preface

Health information processing and applications is one of essential fields in data-driven life health and clinical medicine and it has been highly active in recent decades. The China Health Information Processing Conference (CHIP) is an annual conference held by the Medical Health and Biological Information Processing Committee of the Chinese Information Processing Society (CIPS) of China, with the theme of "Information processing technology helps to explore the mysteries of life, improve the quality of health and improve the level of medical treatment". CHIP is one of leading conferences in the field of health information processing in China and turned into an international event in 2022. It is also an important platform for researchers and practitioners from academia, business and government departments around the world to share ideas and further promote research and applications in this field. CHIP 2022 was organized by the Harbin Institute of Technology (Shenzhen) and the proceedings were published by Springer. Due to the effects of COVID-19, CHIP 2022 conference was held online, whereby people could freely connect to live broadcasts of keynote speeches and presentations.

CHIP 2022 received 35 submissions, of which 14 high-quality papers were selected for publication in this volume after double-blind peer review, leading to an acceptance rate of just 40%. These papers have been categorized into 7 topics: Medical text mining, Gene-Disease semantic association, GDAS track, Medical causal entity and relation extraction, Medical decision tree extraction from unstructured text, OCR of electronic medical documents, and clinical diagnosis coding.

The authors of each paper in this volume reported their novel results of computing methods or application. The volume cannot cover all aspects of Medical Health and Biological Information Processing but may still inspire insightful thoughts for the readers. We hope that more secrets of Health Information Processing will be unveiled, and that academics will drive more practical developments and solutions.

December 2022

Buzhou Tang
Qingcai Chen
Hongfei Lin
Fei Wu
Lei Liu
Tianyong Hao
Yanshan Wang
Haitian Wang

Organization

Honorary Chairs

Hua Xu   UTHealth, USA
Qingcai Chen   Harbin Institute of Technology (Shenzhen), China

General Co-chairs

Hongfei Lin   Dalian University of Technology, China
Fei Wu   Zhejiang University, China
Lei Liu   Fudan University, China

Program Co-chairs

Buzhou Tang   Harbin Institute of Technology (Shenzhen) &
                             Pengcheng Laboratory, China
Tianyong Hao   South China Normal University, China
Yanshan Wang   University of Pittsburgh, USA
Maggie Haitian Wang   Chinese University of Hong Kong, Hong Kong
                             SAR

Young Scientists Forum Co-chairs

Zhengxing Huang   Zhejiang University, China
Yonghui Wu   University of Florida, USA

Publication Co-chairs

Fengfeng Zhou   Jilin University, China
Yongjun Zhu   Yonsei University, South Korea

Evaluation Co-chairs

Jianbo Lei   Medical Informatics Center of Peking University,
                            China
Zuofeng Li   Takeda Co. Ltd., China

Publicity Co-chairs

Siwei Yu   Guizhou Medical University, China
Lishuang Li   Dalian University of Technology, China

Sponsor Co-chairs

Jun Yan   Yidu Cloud (Beijing) Technology Co., Ltd., China
Buzhou Tang   Harbin Institute of Technology (Shenzhen) &
                            Pengcheng Laboratory, China

Web Chair

Kunli Zhang   Zhengzhou University, China

Program Committee

Wenping Guo   Taizhou University, China
Hongmin Cai   South China University of Technology, China
Chao Che   Dalian University, China
Mosha Chen   Alibaba, China
Qingcai Chen   Harbin Institute of Technology (Shenzhen), China
Xi Chen   Tencent Technology Co., Ltd., China
Yang Chen   Yidu Cloud (Beijing) Technology Co., Ltd., China
Zhumin Chen   Shandong University, China
Ming Cheng   Zhengzhou University, China
Ruoyao Ding   Guangdong University of Foreign Studies, China
Bin Dong   Ricoh Software Research Center (Beijing) Co.,
                            Ltd., China
Guohong Fu   Soochow University, China
Yan Gao   Central South University, China
Tianyong Hao   South China Normal University, China

Shizhu He	Institute of Automation, Chinese Academy of Sciences, China
Zengyou He	Dalian University of Technology, China
Na Hong	Digital China Medical Technology Co., Ltd., China
Li Hou	Institute of Medical Information, Chinese Academy of Medical Sciences, China
Yong Hu	Jinan University, China
Baotian Hu	Harbin University of Technology (Shenzhen), China
Guimin Huang	Guilin University of Electronic Science and Technology, China
Zhenghang Huang	Zhejiang University, China
Zhiwei Huang	Southwest Medical University, China
Bo Jin	Dalian University of Technology, China
Xiaoyu Kang	Southwest Medical University, China
Jianbo Lei	Peking University, China
Haomin Li	Children's Hospital of Zhejiang University Medical College, China
Jiao Li	Institute of Medical Information, Chinese Academy of Medical Sciences, China
Jinghua Li	Chinese Academy of Traditional Chinese Medicine, China
Lishuang Li	Dalian University of Technology, China
Linfeng Li	Yidu Cloud (Beijing) Technology Co., Ltd., China
Ru Li	Shanxi University, China
Runzhi Li	Zhengzhou University, China
Shasha Li	National University of Defense Technology, China
Xing Li	Beijing Shenzhengyao Technology Co., Ltd., China
Xin Li	Zhongkang Physical Examination Technology Co., Ltd., China
Yuxi Li	Peking University First Hospital, China
Zuofeng Li	Takeda China, China
Xiangwen Liao	Fuzhou University, China
Hao Lin	University of Electronic Science and Technology, China
Hongfei Lin	Dalian University of Technology, China
Bangtao Liu	Southwest Medical University, China
Song Liu	Qilu University of Technology, China
Lei Liu	Fudan University, China
Shengping Liu	Unisound Co., Ltd., China

Xiaoming Liu	Zhongyuan University of Technology, China
Guan Luo	Institute of Automation, Chinese Academy of Sciences, China
Lingyun Luo	Nanhua University, China
Yamei Luo	Southwest Medical University, China
Hui Lv	Shanghai Jiaotong University, China
Xudong Lv	Zhejiang University, China
Yao Meng	Lenovo Research Institute, China
Qingliang Miao	Suzhou Aispeech Information Technology Co., Ltd., China
Weihua Peng	Baidu Co., Ltd., China
Buyue Qian	Xi'an Jiaotong University, China
Longhua Qian	Suzhou University, China
Tong Ruan	East China University of Technology, China
Ying Shen	South China University of Technology, China
Xiaofeng Song	Nanjing University of Aeronautics and Astronautics, China
Chengjie Sun	Harbin University of Technology, China
Chuanji Tan	Alibaba Dharma Hall, China
Hongye Tan	Shanxi University, China
Jingyu Tan	Shenzhen Xinkaiyuan Information Technology Development Co., Ltd., China
Binhua Tang	Hehai University, China
Buzhou Tang	Harbin Institute of Technology (Shenzhen), China
Jintao Tang	National Defense University of the People's Liberation Army, China
Qian Tao	South China University of Technology, China
Fei Teng	Southwest Jiaotong University, China
Shengwei Tian	Xinjiang University, China
Dong Wang	Southern Medical University, China
Haitian Wang	Chinese University of Hong Kong, China
Haofen Wang	Tongji University, China
Xiaolei Wang	Hong Kong Institute of Sustainable Development Education, Hong Kong SAR
Haolin Wang	Chongqing Medical University, China
Yehan Wang	Unisound Intelligent Technology, China
Zhenyu Wang	South China Institute of Technology Software, China
Zhongmin Wang	Jiangsu Provincial People's Hospital, China
Leyi Wei	Shandong University, China
Heng Weng	Guangdong Hospital of Traditional Chinese Medicine, China

Gang Wu	Beijing Knowledge Atlas Technology Co., Ltd., China
Xian Wu	Tencent Technology (Beijing) Co., Ltd., China
Jingbo Xia	Huazhong Agricultural University, China
Lu Xiang	Institute of Automation, Chinese Academy of Sciences, China
Yang Xiang	Pengcheng Laboratory, China
Lei Xu	Shenzhen Polytechnic, China
Liang Xu	Ping An Technology (Shenzhen) Co., Ltd., China
Yan Xu	Beihang University, Microsoft Asia Research Institute, China
Jun Yan	Yidu Cloud (Beijing) Technology Co., Ltd., China
Cheng Yang	Institute of Automation, Chinese Academy of Sciences, China
Hai Yang	East China University of Technology, China
Meijie Yang	Chongqing Medical University, China
Muyun Yang	Harbin University of Technology, China
Zhihao Yang	Dalian University of Technology, China
Hui Ye	Guangzhou University of Traditional Chinese Medicine, China
Dehui Yin	Southwest Medical University, China
Qing Yu	Xinjiang University, China
Liang Yu	Xi'an University of Electronic Science and Technology, China
Siwei Yu	Guizhou Provincial People's Hospital, China
Hongying Zan	Zhengzhou University, China
Hao Zhang	Jilin University, China
Kunli Zhang	Zhengzhou University, China
Weide Zhang	Zhongshan Hospital Affiliated to Fudan University, China
Xiaoyan Zhang	Tongji University, China
Yaoyun Zhang	Alibaba, China
Yijia Zhang	Dalian University of Technology, China
Yuanzhe Zhang	Institute of Automation, Chinese Academy of Sciences, China
Zhichang Zhang	Northwest Normal University, China
Qiuye Zhao	Beijing Big Data Research Institute, China
Sendong Zhao	Harbin Institute of Technology, China
Tiejun Zhao	Harbin Institute of Technology, China
Deyu Zhou	Southeast University, China
Fengfeng Zhou	Jilin University, China
Guangyou Zhou	Central China Normal University, China
Yi Zhou	Sun Yat-sen University, China

Conghui Zhu	Harbin Institute of Technology, China
Shanfeng Zhu	Fudan University, China
Yu Zhu	Sunshine Life Insurance Co., Ltd., China
Quan Zou	University of Electronic Science and Technology, China
Xi Chen	University of Electronic Science and Technology, China
Yansheng Li	Mediway Technology Co., Ltd., China
Daojing He	Harbin Institute of Technology (Shenzhen), China
Yupeng Liu	Harbin University of Science and Technology, China
Xinzhi Sun	The First Affiliated Hospital of Zhengzhou University, China
Chuanchao Du	Third People's Hospital of Henan Province, China
Xien Liu	Beijing Huijizhiyi Technology Co., Ltd., China
Shan Nan	Hainan University, China
Xinyu He	Liaoning Normal University, China
Qianqian He	Chongqing Medical University, China
Xing Liu	Third Xiangya Hospital of Central South University, China
Jiayin Wang	Xi'an Jiaotong University, China
Ying Xu	Xi'an Jiaotong University, China
Xin Lai	Xi'an Jiaotong University, China

Contents

Healthcare Natural Language Processing

Healthcare Data Mining and Applications

Healthcare Natural Language Processing

Corpus Construction for Named-Entity and Entity Relations for Electronic Medical Records of Cardiovascular Disease

Hongyang Chang[1], Hongying Zan[1,2(✉)], Shuai Zhang[1], Bingfei Zhao[1], and Kunli Zhang[1,2]

[1] School of Computer and Artificial Intelligence, Zhengzhou University, Zhengzhou, Henan, China
iehyzan@zzu.edu.cn
[2] The Peng Cheng Laboratory, Shenzhen, Guangdong, China

Abstract. Electronic medical record (EMR) is an important carrier of medical health information and contains rich knowledge in medical field. Based on the text of EMR of CardioVascular Disease (CVD) and referring to the existing relevant work at home and abroad, this paper formulated the classification system of entities and entity relations and labeling norms suitable for this labeling. The corpus of CardioVascular Disease Electronic Medical Record (CVDEMRC) entity and entity relation is constructed semi-automatically by constructing sentence dictionary and multiple rounds of manual review annotation. The constructed CVDEMRC contains 7,691 named entity concepts and 11,185 entity relations, and both entity and relation have achieved high consistency results, which can provide data basis for CVD research.

Keywords: Cardiovascular disease · Corpus construction · Named entity · Entity relations

1 Introduction

According to the statistics of the Chinese CVD Center[1], from 2005 to 2019, CVD has always accounted for the first cause of death of urban and rural residents in China. CVD has caused a huge burden to society and economy. Therefore, it is necessary to popularize the knowledge of CVD related to the understanding, prevention, discrimination and treatment of the public, weaken the difficulty of obtaining CVD related knowledge, and to reduce the impact of CVD on the families of patients and social.

With the introduction of a series of regulations related to EMR[2], such as "Electronic Medical Record Sharing Document Specification", the rigor, standardization and authenticity of EMRs have been recognized by the public and

Supported by organization x.

[1] https://www.fuwaihospital.org/Sites/Uploaded/File/2021/8/xxgbbg2019.pdf.
[2] http://www.nhc.gov.cn/fzs/s3582h/201609/cf3fe4947766490fbc95a482b47f9112.shtml.

scholars engaged in medical informatization. Therefore, EMRs have gradually become one of the main data sources of clinical medical research. EMRs record all the information of the patient from admission to discharge, which contains a large number of reliable clinical information, including the examination indicators of the patient, treatment methods, changes in the patient's vital signs and medical advice, etc., which can truly reflect the patient's health status and the effect of treatment on the disease. Extracting these information from the EMR text can promote the informatization process of the medical industry, and meet the requirements of the informatization construction of medical institutions with the EMR as the core.

With the implementation of the Healthy China strategy and the construction of electronic medical record informatization, the number of electronic medical records has been increased rapidly. The cost of extracting information from massive medical record text by manual extraction method is expensive and cannot match the speed of new medical record text, so extracting key information from massive data has become the focus of research. Named entity recognition and relation extraction are two important branches in information extraction tasks. Named entity recognition is to identify meaningful entities from given texts, which corresponds to medical texts usually including diseases, symptoms, examinations, parts, surgeries and drugs. The relation extraction task is to extract structured information from unstructured or semi-structured text and represent it in the form of knowledge triples. Limited by the professional characteristics of medical texts, there is a lack of publicly available cardiovascular electronic medical record corpus in Chinese, which hinders the intelligent research of CVD to a certain extent. Therefore, we construct a cardiovascular electronic medical record entity and entity relationship annotation corpus (CVDEMRC). This paper attempts to provide data basis for the related research of CVD information extraction, automatic question answering, intelligent diagnosis and so on.

This paper mainly focuses on the cardiovascular disease electronic medical record text, discusses the determination of the entities contained in the text and the relationship between the entities, proposes the corresponding annotation standard system, and completes the construction of the CVDEMRC.

2   Related Work

At present, many domestic and foreign scholars have focused on corpus construction. In the field of health care, there are well-known medical reference terminology databases SNOMED RT [11] and Clinical Terms Version 3 [7] as well as SNOMED CT [12], which combined these two works and further expanded and updated the clinical standard terminology set of modern western medicine. In 2006, Meystre et al. [5] built a named entity annotation corpus with the size of 160 medical records, including 80 common medical terms, based on medical records such as course records and discharge summaries. In 2008, Savova et al. [10] from Mayo Clinic selected 160 medical records including outpatient records, hospitalization records and discharge summary to construct a named entity corpus of disease entities, and for the first time carefully classified the modification information of entities and entity relationships. In 2009, Roberts et al. [9] constructed a annotated corpus containing 20,000 cancer medical records in order to develop and evaluate a system for automatically extracting important clinical information from medical records, and introduced the construction process of the corpus in detail. Uzuner et al. [14], organizers of the 2010 I2B2 Challenge, published a set of annotated corpus including training set and test set. The corpus was annotated by medical records such as course records and discharge summary, covering three types of entities such as medical problems, examinations and treatments, three types of entity relationships, and six types of information modified for medical problems. In 2013, Mizuki et al. [6] used 50 fictitious Japanese EMRs to construct annotated corpora and used the corpora in the NER task of TCIR-10 MedNLP. In 2017, Leonardo et al. [2] constructed a French-language corpus of medical entities and inter-entity relationships using 500 documents related to medical records, including procedure reports (radiology reports, etc.), discharge summaries, prescriptions, and letters from doctors.

In addition, the construction of Chinese medical corpus started relatively late but has made great progress. In 2013, Lei et al. [4] selected 800 EMRs of Union Hospital, including admission records and discharge summaries, and annotated them by two professional physicians to build a named entity annotation corpus of Chinese EMR. In 2014, Wang et al. [15] collected 11,613 TCM daily clinical records, which were marked by two TCM doctors, and constructed the named entity annotation corpus of TCM clinical medical records. In 2016, Yang et al. [17] collected 992 medical records including the first course record and discharge summary, and constructed a Chinese named entity and entity relationship corpus of EMR. In 2019, Su et al. [13] constructed the first corpus of cardiovascular disease-related risk factors in the Chinese medical field. In 2020, Zan et al. [19–21] built a Chinese symptom knowledge base based on the existing researches on symptom knowledge and combined the characteristics, concepts and the role of symptoms in clinical diagnosis. Using the strategy of deep learning algorithm pre-labeling, they constructed a corpus of pediatric disease entity and entity relationship labeling. The corpus size was more than 2.98 million words, covering 504 kinds of pediatric diseases, and the entity relationship in the corpus was used to build the pediatric medical knowledge map. They also collected multi-source medical texts to complete the corpus annotation of 106 high-incidence diseases. Guan et al. [3] selected medical textbooks, clinical practice guidelines and other texts to construct a Chinese medical information extraction dataset named CMeIE, which contains 11 types of entities and 44 types of entity relationships. In 2021, Ye et al. [18] collected the EMRs of diabetic patients and constructed a corpus of entity and relationship annotation in the electronic medical records of diabetic patients named DEMRC after several rounds of manual annotation.

3   Establishment of Entity and Entity Relationship Labeling System for CVDEMRC

Based on the experience of many works, the entity labeling section defines five types of disease, symptoms, treatment (divided into three categories: surgical treatment, drug treatment and other treatment), examination and body, and four types of entity attribute information representing disease, symptoms, treatment and examination, including modifier information, time information and numerical information (examination results). In the part of entity relationship labeling, based on entity labeling, relationships are divided into 6 types of inter-entity relationships, such as disease and symptom, examination and symptom, treatment and disease, treatment and symptom, body and symptom, and 6 types of entity attribute relationships in attribute information, such as disease and modification, symptom and modification, treatment and modification, disease and time, symptom and time, examination and examination result.

3.1   Disease Entity, Symptom Entity and Their Relationships

Disease refers to the phenomenon that the patient's body is in an abnormal state or causes abnormal life activities due to the disorder of the self-stabilizing regulation. The definition of disease entity mainly corresponds to the International Classification of Diseases (ICD-10) and the part coded as C (Diseases) in the medical thesaurus MeSH, but is not limited to both. In the process of labeling, tools such as medical encyclopedia are also used to determine the entity. Examples of disease entities are as follows:

- No **history of cerebrovascular disease**, no **history of hepatitis, tuberculosis** or **malaria**.
- Preliminary diagnosis: **Chest tightness to be investigated**.
- More than 5 years **post-PCI**.

The definition of symptoms is relatively broad, referring to the discomfort or abnormal reaction of the patient's body, as well as abnormal conditions found through examination. Since ICD-10 did not categorize symptoms clearly, we used the Chinese symptom Knowledge Base [20] and Diagnostics to determine symptom entities in the labeling process. Symptom entity mainly include the patient's own report of abnormal conditions or the family's report on behalf of the patient, doctors through observation, listening, questioning and medical imaging equipment found abnormal conditions of the body. The following are some typical symptom entities in the labeling process:

- No **dizziness, headache, chest pain** and **tightness**.
- There was no **percussion pain** in the left and right renal areas.

Relationship between disease entities and symptom entities: Disease causes symptoms (DCS). Examples are as follows:

– Heart color Ultrasound tips: Left atrial thrombosis after mitral valve replacement. <after mitral valve replacement, DCS, Left atrial thrombosis>
– Now the patient had chest tightness again, and coronary CTA was performed in a local hospital, indicating coronary heart disease. <coronary heart disease, DCS, chest tightness>

3.2   The Treatment Entity and Its Relationships with the Disease Entity and the Symptom Entity

Treatment entity refers to treatment procedures, drug administration and interventions to ameliorate dysregulation, eliminate the cause or relieve symptoms. The labeling process is divided into drug treatment, surgical treatment and other treatment according to the treatment mode.

Drug treatment is mainly defined by the section coded D (Chemicals and Drugs) in the MeSH, the Pharmacology, and drugs that are specified in the medical record as taking certain drugs or listed in the medication guidance. Examples are as follows:

– Medication guidance **Tegafur Gimeracil and Oteracil Potassium Capsule** twice a day, one capsule at a time.
– The patients were given **Biapenem, Mezlocillin sodium/Sulbactam sodium** for anti-infection.

Surgical treatment refers to the process in which doctors use medical instruments such as needle, thread, knife and scissors to cut and suture the patient's body in order to keep the patient in a healthy state. During the labeling process, the surgical treatment entity was determined by referring to the section code E4 (Surgical, Procedures, Operative) in the MeSH, and it was clearly stated in the medical record that the patient underwent certain operations. Note, postoperative should be classified as disease. Examples are as follows:

– The patient underwent **exploratory thoracotomy** for hemothorax.
– **CABG** was performed under general anesthesia.

Other treatment refers to other types of therapy that cannot be determined as drug therapy or surgical therapy, mainly including adjuvant therapy, radiation therapy, chemotherapy and other treatments that indicate the purpose of treatment but do not specify the means and methods of treatment, such as: cardiotonic, diuretic, etc. Examples of other treatment entity are as follows:

– After operation, the patients were treated with **ventilator assisted respiration, antibiotic application, vasoactive drug application, and myocardial nutrition**.
– At the same time, the patients were given symptomatic treatment such as **antiemetic, stomach protection**, and **improving immunity**.

The relationships and examples between the treatment entity and the disease and symptom entities are shown in Table 1

Table 1. The relationships and examples between the treatment entity and the disease entity and the symptom entity. TID/TIS: Treatment improved the disease/symptom. TWD/TWDS: Treatment worsened the disease/symptom. TLD/TLS: Treatment leads to disease/symptom. TAD/TAS: Treatment is applied to disease/symptom.

Relationship	Definition	Example
TID/TIS	Clearly indicate that the disease / symptoms have improved after treatment	Aortic dissection was diagnosed and bentall procedure was performed in our hospital.<bentall procedure, TID, aortic dissection>
TWD/TWS	Treatment of worsening or failing to improve disease / Symptoms	"Cerebral infarction" occurred repeatedly, and aspirin and statins were taken intermittently, with poor effect.<aspirin, TWD, Cerebral infarction><statins, TWD, Cerebral infarction>
TLD/TLS	Diseases / symptoms resulting from the application of treatment	One year earlier, the patient had undergone CABG at this hospital and had developed chest discomfort.<CABG, TLS, chest discomfort>
TAD/TAS	Treatment given to disease / symptoms without mentioning effect	After surgery for adenocarcinoma of the right lung, pemetrexed chemotherapy was given.<pemetrexed, TAD, after surgery for adenocarcinoma of the right lung>

3.3 The Examination Entity and Its Relationships with the Disease Entity and Symptom Entity

Examination entity refers to the examination process, instrument, etc. imposed on the patient to discover or confirm the disease or symptom, so as to assist the doctor to diagnose the patient's condition and formulate treatment plan. For the definition of entity, refer to Medical Imaging [16]. In addition, minor examination items, physiological indicators, body fluid examination and observation made by doctors without the aid of instruments, such as palpation and auscultation, are also marked as examination entities. Examples of some of the more typical checking entities are as follows:

- **Head MRI** showed acute cerebral infarction in the left thalamus.
- **Bilateral babinski sign** was negative. **Murphy sign** was negative.
- The patient had fever yesterday with a **temperature** of 38°C.

The relationships and the examples between the examination entity and the disease entity and the symptom entity are as follows:

1) The examination confirmed the disease.(ECD)
    - 1 month forward gastroscopy indicated "esophageal space occupying lesion" <gastroscopy, ECD, esophageal space occupying lesion>

2) To undergo an examination in order to confirm disease. (UECD)
   - The patient was considered to have acute myocardial infarction and was urgently sent to our hospital for coronary angiography. <coronary angiography, UECD, acute myocardial infarction>
3) The examination confirmed the symptom.(ECS)
   - Electrocardiogram showed sinus rhythm and inverted T wave. <Electrocardiogram, ECS, sinus rhythm>, <Electrocardiogram, ECS, inverted T wave>
4) The examination are taken for symptoms. (EFS)
   - 3 years ago, the child had cyanosis of the lips after movement. Echocardiography at the local hospital showed congenital heart disease. <Echocardiography, EFS, cyanosis of the lips>

3.4   Body Entity and the Relationship to Symptomatic Entity

According to the investigation and analysis of cardiovascular electronic medical records, we found that a large number of body parts and corresponding symptoms are separated by modification information in medical records, and one body part or modifier may correspond to multiple symptoms, such as "thoracic symmetry, no local uplift, collapse, tenderness". The subjects of "symmetry", "local uplift", "collapse" and "tenderness" are all "thoracic", and the word "no", which is used as a negative modifier, isolates the latter part of symptoms from "thoracic". If "thoracic symmetry" and the following are marked separately as symptom entities, then the latter entity lacks the subject and the expression meaning is inconsistent with the original text. For this we added body entity types. Here are some typical examples:

- **Double lungs** breathing sound coarse, no obvious dry-wet rales were heard.
- There was no edema in the **lower limbs**.
- **Moderate tricuspid** and **mitral valve** insufficiency.

Relationship between body entity and symptom entity: Position. Examples are as follows:

- Double lungs breathing sound coarse, not heard and obvious dry-wet rales. <Double lungs, Position, breathing sound coarse>, <Double lungs, Position, dry-wet rales>
- Moderate tricuspid and mitral valve insufficiency. <moderate tricuspid, Position, insufficiency>, <mitral valve, Position, insufficiency>

3.5   Entity Attribute

The attribute information of this annotation includes the modification information of disease entity and symptom entity, the time information of disease entity and symptom entity, and the examination result information.

Modification Information of Entity. The modification information of the entity reflects the relationship between the entity and the patient, mainly reflected in whether the subject of the entity is the patient himself, and the degree, frequency and state of the entity. This information is very important for doctors to understand the patient's condition and for readers to correctly grasp the content of the medical record. Therefore, in order to promote the research progress of information extraction of electronic medical records, we also annotate these modified information in the labeling process. The following are the definitions and examples of modified information.

Modification information of disease and symptom entities fall into eight categories: denial, non-patient, nature, severity, conditional, possible, unconfirmed, and occasional.

1) Denial: The patient himself or the family report, confirm that the patient himself did not happen.
   - **No** history of drug abuse.
   - **Deny** the history of visit prostitutes.
2) Non-patient: Non-patient, but the patient's family.
   - The other **brother** died of cerebral.
   - His **father** had hypertension.
3) Nature: A classification of the state of a disease or symptom.
   - There was a **short paroxysmal** ventricular tachycardia.
   - Atrial septal defect (**secondary hole central type**).
   - The chest pain was **pressor pain**.
4) Severity: Impact on the patient.
   - Pulmonary Hypertension (**Mild**)
   - Hypertension level II is **very high risk**.
5) Conditional: Something that needs to happen under certain circumstances.
   - Chest began six months ago **after exercise**.
6) Possible: cannot be determined with certainty based on current information.
   - Herpes zoster virus infection was **considered** after dermatology consultation.
   - Surgical indications: 1. Aortic dissection**?**
7) Unconfirmed: Likely to happen in the future.
   - There is a **higher risk** of bleeding in the infarct area.
   - There were no postoperative complications and antibiotics were continued to **prevent** infection.
8) Occasional: The occurrence of a disease or symptom that occurs infrequently, as opposed to continuously occurring.
   - **Occasional** atrial premature beats.
   - **Occasionally** sweating profusely, no palpitation and fatigue.

Time Information for the Entity. Whether a patient has suffered from a certain disease or symptom has important reference significance for the current physical condition and clinical diagnosis and treatment, especially hypertension, CABG and other cardiovascular effects are particularly obvious. Therefore, the temporal attribute information of the disease and symptom entities is divided into past and persistent:

1) Past: The patient has occurred in the past and is no longer continuing to occur.
   – Chest pain after intense activity **1 month ago**.
2) persistent: What is currently occurring in the patient, including previous occurrences that continue to the present.
   – Chief complaint: Chest tightness and shortness of breath for **more than 10 days**.
   – Chief complaint: Adenocarcinoma of the left lung **10 months** after surgery.

The Examination Result Information. In the process of labeling, it was found that many examinations in the medical records did not express whether the patient's indicators were in the healthy range in written form, but gave the numerical results of the examination. Although the current deep learning algorithm is not sensitive to numbers and cannot reach the level of logical operation, we believe that these numerical results are direct materials reflecting the patient's situation and may be used in future research. Therefore, we introduce the attribute of examination results, and the examples of examination results are as follows:

– Urine routine test showed glucose **+-**; White blood cell **+-**.
– The test results showed that uric acid was **527μmol/L**.
– Shifting dullness was **negative**.

4 CVDEMRC Construction Process

The corpus construction process is divided into preliminary preparatory work and formal labeling. The overall marking process is shown in Fig. 1

4.1 Preparation

Data Preparation and Processing. The original corpus for the construction of this paper was selected from the electronic medical records of patients in a tertiary hospital in Henan province. The electronic medical records of patients consisted of admission records, medical procedure records, patient assessment, informed documents, surgical records and four other records, and some of the surgical patient records also contained major surgery and unplanned re-operation reports.

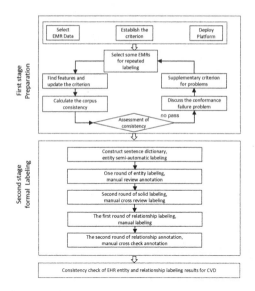

Fig. 1. Flow chart of EMR annotation for CVD

The medical records were analysed and found to contain information about the patient's treatment during his stay in the hospital, including the discharge summary and discharge instructions in the admission record, the medical history and other records. The admission record contains the basic information about the patient at the time of admission, which is the initial status of the patient; the course record includes the first course record and the ward record, which records the examination and treatment received by the patient during the admission and the changes in the patient's condition, which is the process information of the patient; the discharge summary records the basic information of the patient at the time of discharge, which is the end information of the patient's treatment at the admission; and the discharge medical advice contains the information of the medication instruction. We therefore chose these four documents from the medical records as the initial corpus.

Statistical analysis of the raw data revealed that some of the patient record documents collected from hospitals were incomplete, with individual documents missing, so we screened the records and selected 200 complete EMRs for CVD. The screened data is then desensitised, i.e. sensitive information is removed, mainly for de-privacy processing, including the patient's name, telephone number, address, ID number, workplace and doctor's name.

Development and Deployment of Annotation Platform. Based on the above-mentioned labelling system, we developed the labelling specification. The annotation used the entity and entity relationship annotation platform developed by Zhang et al. [22], and was secondarily developed and deployed according to the cardiovascular electronic medical record annotation system. The operating interface of the platform is shown in Fig. 2. The platform is a graphical interface with different entity types marked by different colour blocks and the relationship between two entities indicated by a line and the name of the relationship. In addition, the platform provides progress statistics and annotation comparison reports to improve annotation efficiency and facilitate quality control.

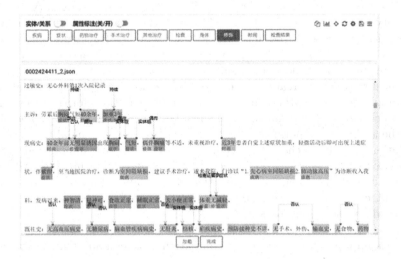

Fig. 2. Entity relationship annotation platform

Training of Tagger. The taggers have involved in the annotation of cardiovascular disease textbook, had some knowledge of the medical field and cardiovascular disease, and were proficient in the use of the annotation platform. In order to become familiar with the markup specifications and improve the quality of the labeling, adaptive pre-markups were conducted prior to formal markups, while issues and situations specific to cardiovascular electronic medical records were identified during the pre-markup process, discussed and the specifications were updated.

4.2 Formal Labeling

After data preparation, specification development, platform deployment and staff training have been completed, the formal annotation of the corpus begins. The formal annotation is divided into 3 parts: semi-automatic annotation of entities, manual review annotation of entities and manual annotation of entity relationships.

Semi-automatic annotation of entities: Observation during pre-labeling revealed that most of the selected EMR files had partial overlap in the description of the medical record, especially in the section on basic patient examination, despite the differences between each patient. Therefore, in order to reduce labour costs and annotation time, we divide the medical record documents according to specific punctuation marks, keeping the same sentence fragment only once as a sentence dictionary, annotating the sentence dictionary with entities by manual annotation, and then automatically annotating all medical record documents by the annotation results of the sentence dictionary.

Entity manual review annotation: Although the constructed sentence dictionary basically covers all the data, the divided sentence fragments only express fragment information and lose information in the sentence and in the context, may result in wrong annotation results due to missing information. In addition, as medical records are created by doctors and are not as rigorously presented as, for example, textbooks, there may be multiple presentations for the same condition, which also causes problems with the labelling after the clauses. Therefore, after the automatic annotation of entities we performed a manual review of the annotation, mainly to check the accuracy of the automatic annotation against the context of the sentence and whether any entities were missing. After the first round of physical manual review, the second round of physical cross review was conducted, that is, the medical records reviewed by the annotators were exchanged for the second review.

Manual annotation of entity relations: Although semi-automatic annotation of entities improves the efficiency of annotation, the semi-automatic annotation method we used for medical record text cannot support entity relation annotation as the annotation of entity relations requires the combination of whole sentences or even cross-sentence information. The relationship annotation process is the same as the entity manual review annotation, i.e. the first round of annotation is carried out by the annotator and the medical record files are exchanged for cross-checking after completion.

5   CVDEMRC's Statistic and Analysis

In order to count the consistency of the annotation, 20 randomly selected charts from each of the cardiology and cardiac surgery charts were annotated for consistency at the end of the formal annotation. Artstein et al. [1] state that the consistency of the annotated corpus is considered to be acceptable when the consistency of the annotated corpus is calculated at 80%. Consistency is calculated as shown in the following equation:

$$P = \frac{A_1 \cap A_2}{A_1} \tag{1}$$

$$R = \frac{A_1 \cap A_2}{A_2} \tag{2}$$

$$F1 = \frac{2 \times P \times R}{P + R} \tag{3}$$

where A_n denotes the annotation result of the n-th annotator and $\cap$ denotes the intersection of the two, in this case the part of the same medical record annotated by both annotators.

Table 2. Corpus consistency and statistics on the number of entities and relationships. Num* indicates the number after removing duplicates.

	Cardiac Surgery		Cardiology		CVD	
	entity	relation	entity	relation	entity	relation
P(%)	96.86	85.92	88.56	79.15	92.86	82.79
R(%)	96.17	87.81	91.92	82.3	94.17	85.29
F(%)	96.51	86.85	90.21	80.69	93.51	84.02
Num	69,090	37,367	81,891	39,447	150,981	76,814
Num*	4,066	5,144	5,087	6,927	7,691	11,185

The corpus annotation consistency results are shown in the upper part of Table 2, with 93.5% consistency in the annotation of named entities and 84.02% consistency in the annotation of entity relationships. The number of entities and entity relationships contained in the corpus is shown in the lower part of Table 2. The consistency shows that the cardiovascular medical record annotation corpus can be recognised. The effectiveness of the proposed method of building a sentence annotation dictionary and semi-automated annotation of entities for medical record type data can be seen from the high consistency of the entities.

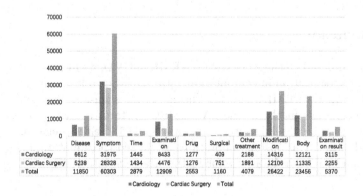

Fig. 3. Statistics on the number of different entities in corpus.

In addition, the cardiology was significantly lower than that of cardiac surgery. According to the number statistics of different entities in Fig. 3, it can be seen that there are more "surgical treatment" entities in the cardiac surgery corpus than in the cardiology, and there are more other types of entities in

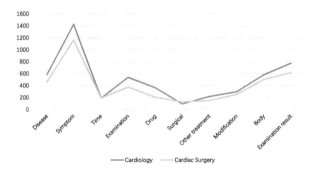

Fig. 4. Comparison of the number of corpus entity categories.

the cardiology department than in the cardiac surgery, especially the symptom, examination and disease entities. This indicates that the information density of electronic medical records in the department of cardiology is relatively high. The number of entities in the different entity types, i.e. the number of de-duplicated entities, is similar to the number of non-de-duplicated entities in Fig. 4, with the exception of "surgical treatment" entities, the number of de-duplicated entities in all entity types being higher in cardiology than in cardiac surgery, indicating a greater diversity of conditions in cardiology. The high density of information, the diversity of disease and symptom and the variety of content presented have caused significant problems in the labelling process, which result in low consistency in the labelling of cardiology records. Since entity relationship annotation is based on the results of entity annotation, the relationship annotation corresponds to the entity annotation situation.

6   Conclusion

In this paper, based on the analysis of the EMR of CVD, we formulated a labeling system and specification in combination with numerous relevant literatures, and constructed the CVDEMRC by using the method of semi-automatic labeling and multi-round review method. The CVDEMRC contains a total of 7,691 named entity concepts (i.e. de-duplicated entities) and 11,185 entity relationships. The entity and entity relationship annotations all passed the annotation consistency test and can provide a data base for further research into CVD.

Experience and Lessons Learned. In this labeling work, after preliminary analysis and investigation, we put forward a semi-automatic labeling method suitable for named entity labeling of EMR. This method improves the labeling efficiency and quality of named entity labeling to a certain extent, but it cannot be applied to entity relationship labeling for the time being. In future work, we would try to conduct the first round of pre-labeling through deep learning algorithm based on the existing medical record corpus, so as to further reduce labor costs and improve labeling efficiency. In addition, our annotation team consisted of 20 computer masters in natural language processing, compared to the annotation group of two annotators by Qu et al. [8] and six annotators by Yang et al. [17], the increase in the number of annotators brought about the problem of difficulty in controlling the quality of annotation. This is also an attempt to use a larger group of annotators to complete a more specialized annotation task in the field, in order to reduce the time cost of corpus construction and to supplement the Chinese medical information extraction corpus with high quality and quickly.

References

1. Artstein, R., Poesio, M.: Inter-coder agreement for computational linguistics. Comput. Linguist. **34**(4), 555–596 (2008)
2. Campillos, L., Deléger, L., Grouin, C., Hamon, T., Ligozat, A.L., Névéol, A.: A French clinical corpus with comprehensive semantic annotations: development of the medical entity and relation Limsi annotated text corpus (merlot). Lang. Resour. Eval. **52**(2), 571–601 (2018)
3. Guan, T., Zan, H., Zhou, X., Xu, H., Zhang, K.: CMeIE: construction and evaluation of chinese medical information extraction dataset. In: Zhu, X., Zhang, M., Hong, Yu., He, R. (eds.) NLPCC 2020. LNCS (LNAI), vol. 12430, pp. 270–282. Springer, Cham (2020). https://doi.org/10.1007/978-3-030-60450-9_22
4. Lei, J., Tang, B., Lu, X., Gao, K., Jiang, M., Xu, H.: A comprehensive study of named entity recognition in Chinese clinical text. J. Am. Med. Inform. Assoc. **21**(5), 808–814 (2014)
5. Meystre, S., Haug, P.J.: Natural language processing to extract medical problems from electronic clinical documents: performance evaluation. J. Biomed. Inform. **39**(6), 589–599 (2006)
6. Morita, M., Kano, Y., Ohkuma, T., Miyabe, M., Aramaki, E.: Overview of the NTCIR-10 MedNLP task. In: NTCIR. Citeseer (2013)
7. O'neil, M., Payne, C., Read, J.: Read codes version 3: a user led terminology. Methods Inf. Med. **34**(01/02), 187–192 (1995)
8. Qu, C., Guan, Y., Yang, J., Zhao, Y., Liu, Y.: Construction of Chinese electronic medical record named entity annotation corpus. High Technol. Lett. **2**, 143–150 (2015)
9. Roberts, A., et al.: Building a semantically annotated corpus of clinical texts. J. Biomed. Inform. **42**(5), 950–966 (2009)
10. Savova, G.K., et al.: Mayo clinical text analysis and knowledge extraction system (cTAKES): architecture, component evaluation and applications. J. Am. Med. Inform. Assoc. **17**(5), 507–513 (2010)
11. Spackman, K.A., Campbell, K.E., Côté, R.A.: SNOMED RT: a reference terminology for health care. In: Proceedings of the AMIA annual fall symposium, p. 640. American Medical Informatics Association (1997)
12. Stearns, M.Q., Price, C., Spackman, K.A., Wang, A.Y.: SNOMED clinical terms: overview of the development process and project status. In: Proceedings of the AMIA Symposium, p. 662. American Medical Informatics Association (2001)
13. Su, J., et al.: Cardiovascular disease risk factor labeling system and corpus construction based on chinese electronic medical records. Acta Automatica Sinica **45**(2) (2019)

14. Uzuner, Ö., South, B.R., Shen, S., DuVall, S.L.: 2010 i2b2/VA challenge on concepts, assertions, and relations in clinical text. J. Am. Med. Inform. Assoc. **18**(5), 552–556 (2011)
15. Wang, Y., et al.: Supervised methods for symptom name recognition in free-text clinical records of traditional Chinese medicine: an empirical study. J. Biomed. Inform. **47**, 91–104 (2014)
16. Wu, E.: Medical imaging fifth edition (2003)
17. Yang, J., et al.: Construction of named entity and entity relationship corpus for Chinese electronic medical records. J. Softw. **11**, 2725–2746 (2016)
18. Ye, Y., Hu, B., Zhang, K., Zan, H.: Construction of corpus for entity and relation annotation of diabetes electronic medical records. In: Proceedings of the 20th Chinese National Conference on Computational Linguistics, pp. 622–632 (2021)
19. Zan, H., et al.: Construction of Chinese medical knowledge map based on multisource text. J. Zhengzhou Univ. (Science Edition) **52**(2), 45–51 (2020)
20. Zan, H., Han, Y., Fan, Y., Niu, C., Zhang, K., Sui, Z.: Establishment and analysis of Chinese symptom knowledge base. J. Chin. Inf. **34**(4), 30–37 (2020)
21. Zan, H., Liu, T., Niu, C., Zhao, Y., Zhang, K., Sui, Z.: Construction and application of named entity and entity relationship annotation corpus for pediatric diseases. J. Chin. Inf. **34**(5), 19–26 (2020)
22. Zhang, K., Zhao, X., Guan, T., Shang, B., Li, Y., Zan, H.: Construction and application of medical text oriented entity and relationship annotation platform. J. Chin. Inf. **34**(6), 117–125 (2020)

Hybrid Granularity-Based Medical Event Extraction in Chinese Electronic Medical Records

Shuangcan Xue, Jintao Tang[✉], Shasha Li, and Ting Wang

School of Computer, National University of Defense Technology, Changsha, China
{xuescan,tangjintao,shashali,tingwang}@nudt.edu.cn

Abstract. Chinese medical event extraction (CMEE) has risen the attention of a large amount of researchers. The event extraction in Chinese electronic medical records (CEMRs) has been an important aspect of EMRs information extraction. Most recent work solves the CMEE task, either by a pre-training language model and ensemble, or performing data augmentation through generating dummy data. In this work, we present a hybrid-granularity approach for CMEE task, and obtain a 3.46% absolute improvement in the F1-score over previous models with the same condition of low resource in trainingdata. Our approach essentially builds on a hybrid granularity-based extracter and a multi-rule ensembler based on medical feature word according to the characteristics of the data itself. Shown by the results, our extracter can extract more rightful tumor-related attributes from different granularities of data by reducing the harmful noise from useless sentences of original clinical text. Moreover, the results show that the multi-rule ensembler based medical feature word efficiently solves the problem of Chinese medical entities de-duplication and boundary ambiguity.

Keywords: Medical event extraction · Hybrid granularity · Medical feature words

1 Introduction

With the rapid spread of electronic medical records and the arrival of the medical big data era, how to efficiently and automatically extract rightful and useful information from vast amounts of CEMRs for patients to know their condition or for doctors to do scientific research has risen many researchers' attention. The MEE in CMERs has been an important aspect of EMR information extraction. MEE is a crucial and challenging task in medical information extraction in Chinese. In the medical area, event extraction is mainly used to convert unstructured text records into structured and clear event data. It extracts various elements of events in the origin data to form structured information, which can be applied to information retrieval, knowledge graph construction, intelligent question answering, etc. It is also convenient for doctors directly to use these substantial structured data to carry out related medical research, saving their time and energy.

© The Author(s), under exclusive license to Springer Nature Singapore Pte Ltd. 2023
B. Tang et al. (Eds.): CHIP 2022, CCIS 1772, pp. 19–36, 2023.
https://doi.org/10.1007/978-981-19-9865-2_2

CCKS 2019 organized a Chinese medical event extraction (CMEE) task, which defines three attributes of tumor events, including tumor patient's tumor primary site, primary tumor size, and metastatic sites. The three attributes of tumor events are defined as follows:

- **Tumor Primary Site**: The body site of the primary tumor, as distinct from metastatic sites;
- **Primary Tumor Size**: describing the measurement of the length, area or volume of the primary tumor;
- **Tumor Metastasis Site**: the metastatic site of the primary tumor. Theoretically, the tumor can metastasize to any other part of the body except the primary site of the tumor.

We need to identify and extract these attributes about a tumor event from CMERs generated from real medical scenarios. As we can see in an example from Fig. 1, the three attributes of a tumor event in an electronic medical record are "右肺下叶", "17 × 15 MM" and "左肺上叶". The corpus provided by organizers includes 1000 entries of manually annotated CEMRs as training data, and 400 entries of raw CEMRs as test data. These models solving the CMEE task mainly focus on the pre-training language model, ensemble and data augmentation [14–16, 21]. Although the event extraction ability has been improved to a certain extent, their approaches take little account of data characteristics and the connection of medical event attributes.

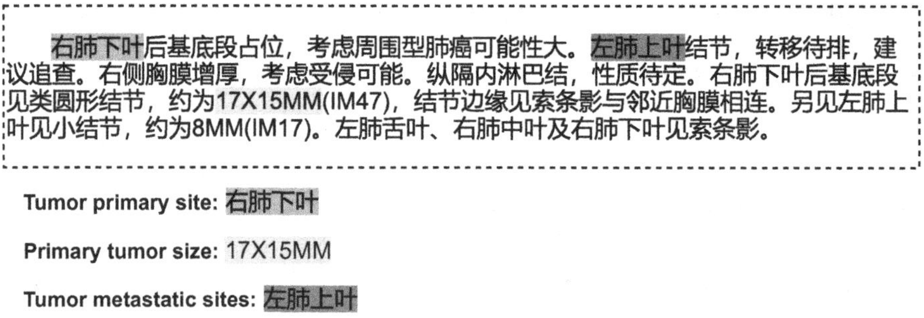

> 右肺下叶后基底段占位，考虑周围型肺癌可能性大。左肺上叶结节，转移待排，建议追查。右侧胸膜增厚，考虑受侵可能。纵隔内淋巴结，性质待定。右肺下叶后基底段见类圆形结节，约为17X15MM(IM47)，结节边缘见索条影与邻近胸膜相连。另见左肺上叶见小结节，约为8MM(IM17)。左肺舌叶、右肺中叶及右肺下叶见索条影。

Tumor primary site: 右肺下叶

Primary tumor size: 17X15MM

Tumor metastatic sites: 左肺上叶

Fig. 1. An example of a part of a Chinese medical record in real scenarios. Different attributes of tumor event are distinguished by colored rounded rectangles and are listed below.

We found some features about the corpus by doing a preliminary statistical analysis of data as follows:

- The length of CMERs varies.The longest is more than 1600 words and the shortest is only about 100 words. But the attributes distribution across sentences, which may result in longer text and more noise from the usless sentences;

- The three attributes of tumor event may be incomplete in one CMER;
- Primary tumor size depends on the tumor primary site. In general, primary tumor size and tumor primary site coexist at the multi-sentences level in the CEMR;
- Tumor metastatic site and tumor primary site are body parts, which can be extract in a single sentence in Chinese.

To this end, this paper proposes a hybrid granularity-based extraction framework to achieve the CMEE task based on the above analysis, which avoids the limitation of the single-granularity model extraction performance. This framework consists of two crutial parts, as shown in Fig. 2.

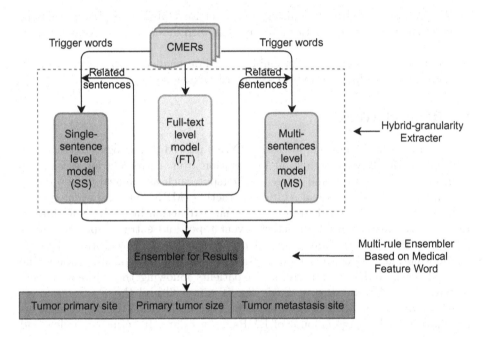

Fig. 2. The whole framework of our approach.

In the first stage of the framework, a hybrid-granularity extracter is proposed to extract more candidate tumor event attributes entities to improve the overall recall rate, which consists of three models with the same architecture, including single-sentence level (SS), multi-sentence level (MS) and full-text level (FT). We use FT to extract the all tumor event attributes. Meanwhile, we can get the attributes entities distribution information for the tag sequence. Then we combine related sentences into a new input for SS and MS by the distribution information. The SS mainly extract tumor metastatic site and tumor primary site. The MS mainly extract primary tumor size as a supplement for FT. The difference among the three models are the granularity of the training data and the target attributes. We use data of different granularities to train the same model to obtain different extraction capabilities, which improves the recall rate and the transferability of the extracter for more CMERs in different scenarios. On the one hand, we can reduce harmful noise from usless sentences for SS and MS by the new input combined with related sentences according to the FT. On the other hand, it helps us get a higher recall rate by the hybrid-granularity extracter. In the second stage, we introduce a multi-rules ensembler based on medical feature word to remove repetition and directly select more reasonable event entities from candidate entities. We build a medical feature word dictionary, automatically label each candidate site, and then remove duplicated entities to improve the precision rate.

The main contribution of this paper can be summarized as follows:

- We proposed a hybrid-granularity extracter for CMEE task. Using different granularity of training data obtain models with different extraction capabilities;
- We introduce a multi-rules ensembler based on medical feature word to integrate those results from hybrid-granularity extracter;

2   Related Works

How to use natural language processing (NLP) related technologies to efficiently and automatically extract helpful information from extremely large amounts of medical texts has become a research hotspot, such as medical named entity recognition (MNER), medical relation extraction (MRE), medical event extraction (MEE), etc. Among them, medical event extraction in EMRs is an important research direction, which detects event types and extracts specified event attributes from unstructured medical text to realize the structuring of medical information. EMRs are the descriptive recorded by medical staff around the medical needs and service activities of patients following the relevant writing regulations in *Medical Record Basic Specification* [2] and the *Basic Specifications for Electronic Medical Records(Trial)* [1]. At the same time, the hospitals also have stored a large amount of EMRs as raw data. In terms of models and methods, deep learning and neural networks have become mainstream.

The English medical events extraction task is relatively early compared to the Chinese. Represented by i2b2 (Informatics for Integrating Biology & the Bedside) and SemEval (International Workshop on Semantic Evaluation), many evaluations have been organized, such as i2b2 2012 shared task [3], SemEval-2015 task6 [4], SemEval-2016 task12 [5], SemEval-2017 task12 [6], etc., mainly to extract event information from the electronic medical records and pathological reports of cancer patients. In the field of English medical event extraction, there have a lot of related work been done. In 2020, Ramponi [7] et al. firstly introduced Biomedical Event Extraction as Sequence Labeling (BEESL), which outperformed the best system on the Genia 2011 benchmark by 1.57% absolute F1-score reaching 60.22% and made it a viable approach for large-scale real-world scenarios. Huang [8] et al. proposed to incorporate domain knowledge to a pre-trained language model via a hierarchical graph representation encoded by

Graph Edge-conditioned Attention Networks (GEANet), which achieved 1.41% F1-score and 3.19% F1-score improvements on all events and complex events on BioNLP 2011 GENIA Event Extraction task. Li [9] et al. propose a novel knowledge base (KB)-driven tree-structured long short-term memory networks (Tree-LSTM) framework, which effectively solves the problem of encoding contextual information and external background knowledge.

In recent years, The China Conference on Health Information Processing (CHIP) and the China Conference on Knowledge Graph and Semantic Computing (CCKS) have begun to organize evaluation tasks for clinical medical event extraction, such as CHIP 2018 task 1 [10], CCKS2019 task 1 [11], CCKS2020 task 3 [12], CHIP2021 task 2 [13], etc. Ji [14] et al. proposed a multi neural networks based approach, which consists of a couple of BiLSTM-CRF models and a CNN model for sentence classification, and obtained 76.35% F1-score on the official test dataset on CCKS2019 task 1. Dai [15] et al. completed the training of domain adaptation and task adaptation based on the pre-trained language model RoBERTa, superimposed the conditional random field (CRF) on the basis of the RoBERTa model Transformer encoder for sequence labeling, and completed the small sample condition. It achieved the best F1-score of 76.23% on CCKS2020 task 3. Gan [16] et al. proposed a combination strategy of unsupervised text mode enhancement and label mode enhancement based on the pre-training model, which makes full use of the limited labeled data and unlabeled data in the dataset to improve the generalization ability of the model. Ji [22] et al. First applied the BiLSTM-CRF model to medical NER on Chinese EMRs. Then the attention mechanism is added to the BiLSTM-CRF model to construct the attention, aiming at alleviating the problem of label inconsistency.

3 Method

The proposed approach mainly consists of two components: the **hybrid-granularity extracter** for the attributes of tumor event extraction and the **multi-rule ensembler based on medical feature word** for integrating the results from the extracter. The framework of our approach is illustrated in Fig. 2.

3.1 Hybrid-Granularity Extracter

We take into account the incompleteness of event attributes and the correlation between attributes in an EMR. Primary tumor size depends on the tumor primary site. In general, primary tumor size and tumor primary site coexist at the multi-sentences level in the CEMR. So we introduce the multi-sentence level model (MS) to extract primary tumor size and tumor primary site. Moreover, there is no strict or clear link between tumor metastatic site and tumor primary site, because that the tumor primary site is a specific body part or organ, and tumor metastatic site maybe any other part of the body with more than one in number. But what they have in common is that they're both body parts. More importantly, we can extract the tumor metastatic site or tumor primary site from a single sentence. So we introduce the single-sentence level model (SS) to extract tumor metastatic site and tumor primary site.

Procedure 1. The process of the hybrid-granularity extracter

Input: X: CMERs
Output: Y: The atrributes entities of mdeical events in CMERs
 1: Given full-text level model FT, multi-sentence level model MS, single-sentence level model SS and the list of trigger words for SS or MS: T.
 2: **for** each $i \in [1, |X|]$ **do**
 3:     $AE_{FT}=$ attributes entities in the result of X_i in FT
 4:     $RS_{SS}=$ relevant attributes sentences for SS according to AE_{FT}(including tumor metastatic site and tumor primary site)
 5:     $RS_{MS}=$ relevant attributes sentences for MS according to AE_{FT}(including tumor primary site and primary tumor size)
 6:     $TS=$ sentences in X_i triggered by T
 7:     $input_{SS}= RS_{SS} + TS$
 8:     $input_{MS}= RS_{MS} + TS$
 9:     $AE_{SS}=$ attributes entities in the result of $input_{SS}$ in SS
10:     $AE_{MS}=$ attributes entities in the result of $input_{MS}$ in MS
11:     $Y_i= AE_{FT} + AE_{SS} + AE_{MS}$
12: **end for**
13: **return** Y

Full-text Level Model (FT). FT takes the full text of an EMR as input to extract three attributes of tumor event including tumor primary site, primary tumor size and tumor metastatic site, which is the subject of the extraction framework. The architecture of FT is shown in Fig. 3 The first part of the FT is PCL-MedBERT [18] as the character embedding layer to obtain the sentence representation, i.e. $X = (x_1, x_2..., x_n)$, where $x_i \in R^d$, and d is word embedding dimension. The second part of the FT is the transformer encoder consisting of two encoder layers. Then the result is fed into a BiLSTM encoder in which the forward LSTM computes a representation of the sequence $(\overrightarrow{h_1}, \overrightarrow{h_2} ..., \overrightarrow{h_n})$ from left to right, and the backward one $(\overleftarrow{h_1}, \overleftarrow{h_2} ..., \overleftarrow{h_n})$ computes in reverse , generating the representation of every word in the sentence $(h_1, h_2..., h_n) \in R^{n \times m}$ by concatenating the word's left and right context representations $h_i = [\overrightarrow{h_i}, \overleftarrow{h_i}] \in R^m$. Then a linear layer is set to map the hidden state vector from m-dimension to k-dimension (k is the number of tags defining in the tagging set), and then we get a output matrix $P = (p_1, p_2..., pn) \in R^{n \times k}$ from the BiLSTM layer. Each element p_{ij} of $P \in R^{n \times k}$ can be regarded as the probability that tag the word x_i with the j_{th} tag. The last is a CRF [11] layer to find the final sequence path. The parameter of CRF layer is a transition matrix A with a dimension of $(k+2) \times (k+2)$, where k is tag number, and A_{ij} represents the transition score from the tag i to the tag j. Then we can use A and P to calculate the score for the a sentence X and a tag sequence $y = (y_1, y_2...y_n)$ by the following formula:

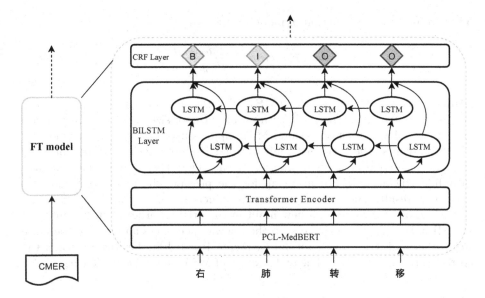

Fig. 3. The network architecture of model. (FT, MS and SS have same network architecture)

$$s(X, y) = \sum_{i=0}^{n} A_{y_i, y_{i+1}} + \sum_{i=1}^{n} P_{i, y_i} \tag{1}$$

We can see that the score(X, y) equals the sum of scores of all words in sentence decided by the transition matrix A and the matrix P described above. And then normalize by Softmax to get the conditional probability, as shown in following formula:

$$P(y|X) = \frac{exp(s(X, y))}{\sum_{y'} exp(s(X, y'))} \tag{2}$$

The goal of CRF layer is to have the highest probability that the input X corresponds to the correct sequence y, which is expressed by the likelihood function as follows:

$$\log(P(y|X)) = s(X, y) - \log(\sum_{y'} exp(s(X, y'))) \tag{3}$$

During the encoding process, we can get the optimal tag path by Viterbi algorithm with dynamic planning, as the following formula shows.

$$y^* = \arg\max_{y'} s(X, y') \tag{4}$$

Then we use the loss function of model as following:

$$LossFunction = \frac{P_{RealPath}}{P_{TotalPath}} \tag{5}$$

Multi-sentence Level Model (MS). We use MS to extract primary tumor size as a supplement to the EMR with primary tumor size and no primary tumor size in the FT's extraction results. MS's input consists of two parts. One part is the sentences where the attributes(primary tumor size and tumor primary site) are located from FT's extraction result. The other part is the sentences including trigger words to make up for the possible shortcomings from FT's extraction result. The trigger words mainly include "癌" , "MT", "转移" and "恶性" . Then we compose a new input in the original order of these sentences in EMRs. By this way, can we keep the relevant sentences and reduce the noise from other useless sentences for our extracter. It is helpful for MS to extract the correct attributes entities. The architecture of MS is the same of FT (see Fig. 3).

Single-sentence Level Model (SS). We use SS to extract the attributes(tumor metastatic site and tumor primary site) as a supplement to the EMR in the FT's extraction results. SS's input also consists of two parts. One part is the sentences where the attributes are located from FT's extraction result. The other part is the sentences including trigger words to make up for the possible shortcomings from FT's extraction result, which are same with the MS's trigger words. The architecture of SS is the same of FT(see Fig. 3).

3.2   Multi-rule Ensembler Based on Medical Feature Words

The result of extracter is the sum from FT, SS and MS. The candidates of primary tumor size consist of the results of FT and MS. But the MS only extract from these CMERs that there is no primary tumor size in the result of FT. So there is not duplicate candidate in this attribute. Tumor primary site and tumor metastatic site consist of the results from FT and SS. We designed SS to extract more rightful entities as a supplemnt for FT. Therefore, it is inevitable to introduce duplicate data in this process. So we need to intergrate the result from the hybrid-granularity extracter. Moreover, we found that all body parts contain one or more special and uncommon words in Chinese, which can be used as a label for classification or to determine whether it is a body part. Such as the "胃" (stomach) in "胃癌" (gastric cancer), ("肝" (liver), "叶" (lobe))in "肝脏左叶" (left lobe of the liver), etc. We called them medical feature words. Finally, we designed a multi-rule ensembler based on medical feature words.

This component's main work are deduplication and the correction of format in tumor primary site and tumor metastatic site from the result of the extracter. We label candidate body parts with medical feature words in extraction results, and then utilize some rules to remove duplicate results and correct the output format particularly in tumor metastatic site.

Tumor Primary Site. We use the multi-rule ensembler based on medical feature words for tumor primary site to deduplicate based on the following considerations:

1. There may be one tumor primary site or more than one in a patient's EMR;
2. A tumor primary site may have multiple candidates from the hybrid-granularity extracter in our method, which need us to select a more reasonable as the attribute value;
3. The number of common tumor types is limited and a tumor event basically has only one primary site.

So we firstly build a light dictionary D_{TPS} based on medical feature word for tumor primary sites, which helps us to automatically label each candidate. The light dictionary consists of 14 common elements including "肺" , "胃" , "鼻咽" , etc.(See appendix for details) And then we use these labels to do classification by some sample rules to solve the first question. For example, we use "胃" (stomach) from "胃癌" (gastric cancer) as the feature word of "胃窦" , "肺" (lung) from "肺癌" (lung cancer) as the feature word of "左肺" (left lung) or "右肺门" (hilum of the right lung) and so on. Meanwhile, we can add or delete related feature words to the light dictionary according to medical needs. Another important reason we do this is that a tumor event basically has only one primary site. Then we follow the steps below to deduplicate for tumor primary site candidates:

1. Labeling each candidate by using medical feature words, which can remove some non-body part words and classify the candidates according to the label;
2. Selecting one more reasonable candidate as the output in each category from the step 1 by the following rules:
   R1. Selecting the candidate that is closer to primary tumor size;
   R2. Selecting the candidate that is closer to the "癌" (cancer), "MT", "病灶" (lesion) or "CA" if there is no primary tumor size in the CMER.

We use the medical feature-words dictionary to label each candidate and select more reasonable by rules, which efficiently solves the problem of deduplication for tumor primary site.

Tumor Metastatic Site. We use the multi-rule ensembler based on medical feature words for tumor metastatic site to deduplicate candidate answers and correct the format based on the following considerations:

1. There are basically multiple entities for tumor metastatic site in a tumor event;
2. A entity may have multiple candidates from the hybrid-granularity extracter in our method, which need us to select more reasonable one;
3. A candidate entity from the hybrid-granularity extracter may be split into multiple entities in the final output.

Firstly, we use the tag sequence information from the extracter to obtain the real location index of the entities. If entities are overlapping or adjacent, separated by "、", then we have reason to believe that these need to combined into one entity. Then we will get some single entities and strings consisting of multiple entities, which achieves the purpose of partial deduplication and alleviation of boundary ambiguity. Lastly, we use some easy rules to segment the strings into entities and the dictionary D_{TMS} based on medical feature word to judge whether an entity is a part of the body. We design a decomposition algorithm for the strings consisting of multiple entities segmenting into entities (See appendix for details).

Then we follow the steps below to deduplicate candidate answers and correct the format for for tumor metastatic site:

1. Combining these overlapping or adjacent entities into a string by the tag sequence information from the extracter;
2. Removing the invalid candidate and correcting the left boder by the following rules:
   R1. Remove the candidate if the candidate does not contain any medical feature word in D_{TMS} ;
   R2. Take advantage of the speciality of the first character to correct the left boder, which is that the first character at the left boundary of the entity must be a Chinese word or a medical feature word.
   R3. Feed the strings in the step 1 into the decomposition algorithm, which help us automatically segment these strings into multiple entities.

4   Experiments

This section introduces **the data pre-processing, experimental setup** and **evaluation and results**.

4.1   Data Pre-processing

There are some special characters in the original CMERs, which is harmful for the extracter to learn from texts. So we firstly clean the training dataset by deleting these illegal characters and converting English punctuation into Chinese. Meanwhile, the training dataset directly provides corresponding answers for the attributes of tumor events, not the position index. We also need to label the location of answers in the data.

Data Cleaning. This step aims to remove illegal characters from the official evaluation data and normalize them. Specific cleaning strategies include:

1. Convert English punctuation into Chinese, such as '.' and 'o';
2. Remove special characters, such as spaces, '_x0004_', etc.

Data Annotation. The training dataset directly provides corresponding answers for the attributes of tumor events, not the position index. Our extraction system uses the sequence labeling(BIO) model to solve this task, and it needs to mark the position of the attributes in the origin EMRs. Generally, the answer position is directly marked back by exact matching. For the case where a small number of candidates fail to match, or multiple candidates are matched need to label these by ourselves.

Text Segmentation. In this step, the length of some EMRs is too long to directly as the input for the pre-training model(MCBERT), which needs to segment these EMRs to ensure that the length of text segment does not exceed 510 characters. At the same time, we also make sure of the integrity of the sentence. We use two-way segmenting forward and backward, taking sentences as the unit so as to meet the requirements.

4.2 Experimental Setup

Our models are implemented in PyTorch with python 3.6. The version of torch is 1.8.0. All experiments are conducted on a 6-core CPU machine and NVIDIA RTX 3060 with CUDA 11.2. During the process of model training, we used the PCL-MedBERT from Peng Cheng Lab as the embedding layer, and we used Adam as the optimizer withthe learning rate to 2e–5 to optimize the output layer of the PCL-MedBERT. The dimension of a token is 768. The other parts in our framework used Adam as the optimizer withthe learning rate to 2e–4. In the part of transformer encoder, the heads of multi-head attention is 3 and the dropout is 0.2. The training epoch of the experiment is 100, and the batch-size is 8.

We evaluate the proposed method on the CCKS2019 MEE task test dataset compared with the SOTA in the CCKS2019. The result is shown in Table 2. We further introduce several variants of our method by excluding the single-sentence level model (named Method/SS), multi-sentences level model (named Method/MS) and the ensembler for intergrating result (named Method/ER) to validate their impacts in an individual and combination manner. We also introduce the baseline of our method, which removes SS, MS and ER. We don't set the variant of our method by excluding the full-text level model (named Method/FT) because that the inputs of SS and MS depend on the result of the model FT. These results are shown in Table 3.

4.3   Evaluation and Results

Evaluation Metrics. Since multiple entities may appear in one attribute of tumor event in each EMR, the evaluation metrics use all of the entities of three attributes extracted rather than three attribute values to calculate precision and recall. A simple statistical profile of the dataset in given in Table 1.

In the next section, for better understanding, we give the micro-average precisions (P), recalls (R) and F1-scores (F1) of three attributes, respectively.

$$P = \frac{TP}{TP + FP} \tag{6}$$

$$R = \frac{TP}{TP + FN} \tag{7}$$

$$F1 = \frac{2 \times P \times R}{P + R} \tag{8}$$

Table 1. Statistical characterization of the dataset used in our experiments.

Category	Entity number in train data	Entity number in test data
Tumor primary site	1002	290
Primary tumor size	513	107
Tumor metastasis site	2134	473
Overall	3649	870

Results and Discussion. The results of three attributes in our models on the CCKS2019 MEE task's test dataset are reported in Table 2. According to Table 2, it can be seen that we got the integral F1-score of three attributes is 79.81%, using our approach, which has a 3.46% absolute improvement in F1-score compared with the SOTA in CCKS2019. What's more, Our overall model has a better ability to extract primary tumor size, followed by tumor primary site and tumor metastatic sites, which also shows that the extraction of tumor metastatic sites is more complicated.

Table 2. Testing results of our approach on the dataset released by CCKS 2019.

Category	P(%)	R(%)	F1(%)
Tumor primary site	78.69	81.75	80.19
Primary tumor size	88.31	92.45	90.33
Tumor metastasis site	74.66	72.12	73.37
Overall	**79.51**	**80.11**	**79.81**
The SOTA in CCKS2019	-	-	76.35

Table 3. The performance of different variants of our method in MEE task.

Model	Tumor primary site			Primary tumor size			Tumor metastatic site			Overall
	P(%)	R(%)	F1(%)	P(%)	R(%)	F1(%)	P(%)	R(%)	F1(%)	F1(%)
Method	78.69	81.75	**80.19**	88.31	92.45	90.33	74.66	72.12	**73.37**	**79.81**
Method/SS	75.24	76.16	75.70	88.81	92.49	**90.61**	74.80	67.30	70.85	77.87
Method/MS	78.16	81.02	79.57	87.31	90.00	88.64	74.66	72.12	**73.37**	79.20
Method/ER	60.82	87.19	71.66	88.31	92.45	90.33	63.27	73.16	67.85	74.03
Baseline	66.32	77.02	71.27	87.06	89.74	88.39	71.29	66.57	68.85	74.74

By comparing Method with Method/SS, we can see that we obtain 4.59% and 4.82% improvement in recall rate about tumor primary site and tumor metastatic site since SS effectively provides more correct candidate entities. By comparing Method with Method/MS, MS also provides an effective supplement in primary size. The multi-rules ensembler based on medical feature word gains a 5.78% improvement in overall F1-score, which proves the effectiveness of our method. The last but not least, we can see that our method obtain a 5.07% improvement in overall F1-score by comparing Method with Baseline, which proves that the improvement comes from our method again.

5 Conclusion

In this paper, we introduce the hybrid granularity-based approach that achieves better results in the CCKS2019 MEE task under the condition of small samples by a hybrid-granularity extracter, which extracts more rightful tumor-related attributes from different granularities of data by reducing the negative noise from useless sentences of origin clinical text. It obtained 79.81% F1-score with a 3.46% absolute improvement compared with the SOTA in CCKS2019. Moreover, the results showed that the designed multi-rule ensembler is efficient for solving the problem of Chinese medical entity deduplication and boundary ambiguity. After data analysis, we found that the ability to extract in tumor metastatic sites needs to be enhanced in the future.

Acknowledgements. We would like to thank CCKS for organizing the MEE task and Yidu Cloud (Beijing) Technology Co., Ltd. for providing the original dataset in the study.

A   Appendix

A.1   Medical Feature Words

We use the special word in the body parts as medical feature words to label each candidate or to determine the entity whether it is a body part in the multi-rule ensembler. The medical feature words mainly consist of two parts:the D_{TPS} for tumor primary site and D_{TMS} for tumor metastatic site. The D_{TPS} is a light dictionary based on medical feature words for tumor primary site, which is extracted manually from the tumor primary site in training dataset as follow:

$$D_{TPS} = [\text{"胃"}, \text{"肠"}, \text{"肝"}, \text{"鼻咽"}, \text{"肺"}, \text{"膀胱"}, \text{"卵巢"}, \text{"宫"}, \text{"乳"}, \text{"左肾"}, \text{"右肾"}, \text{"肾盂"}, \text{"食管"}, \text{"胸"}]$$

We realize the classification of all candidates from the tumor primary site by this light dictionary, and select more reasonable one in each category. The D_{TMS} based on medical feature words for tumor metastatic site, which is is extracted manually from the body parts by searching in the Baidu Encyclopedia as follow:

$D_{TMS} = [\text{"椎"}, \text{"骨"}, \text{"腋"}, \text{"肋"}, \text{"关节"}, \text{"腱"}, \text{"口"}, \text{"牙"},$
$\text{"舌"}, \text{"腺"}, \text{"腰"}, \text{"咽"}, \text{"食"}, \text{"胃"}, \text{"肠"}, \text{"肝"}, \text{"脏"}, \text{"胆"},$
$\text{"囊"}, \text{"膜"}, \text{"鼻"}, \text{"腔"}, \text{"喉"}, \text{"肺"}, \text{"膈"}, \text{"肾"}, \text{"管"}, \text{"膀胱"},$
$\text{"道"}, \text{"卵巢"}, \text{"子宫"}, \text{"睾"}, \text{"心"}, \text{"脉"}, \text{"淋"}, \text{"髓"}, \text{"胸"}, \text{"脾"},$
$\text{"体"}, \text{"神"}, \text{"经"}, \text{"脑"}, \text{"脊"}, \text{"眼"}, \text{"耳"}, \text{"骨"}, \text{"乳"}, \text{"叶"},$
$\text{"焦"}, \text{"腑"}, \text{"颞"}, \text{"颈"}, \text{"L"}, \text{"T"}, \text{"C"}, \text{"S"}]$

The D_{TMS} is mainly used to determine if an candidate entity is a body part.

A.2   The Decomposition Algorithm

We designed a decomposition algorithm to correct the format of the attributes entities about tumor metastatic site as shown in Algorithm 2.

Algorithm 2 The decomposition algorithm

Input: $S = (s_1, s_2...s_n)$: The string consisting of phrases s_i which are linked by ',' in Chinese.

Output: $E = (e_1, e_2...e_m)$: The multiple entities of tumor metastatic site in S

1: Given labels for s_i as following:

$L1.$: "结节" or "淋巴结" in s_i;
$L2.$: the first and last character of s_i are Chinese word;
$L3.$: the first is a Chinese word and last character of s_i is not a Chinese word;
$L4.$: the first and last character of s_i are not Chinese word;
$L5.$: the s_i is a body part judged by D_{TMS} ;
$L6.$: the s_i is not a body part judged by D_{TMS} ;
  (The above tags are in descending order of priority and each phrase s_i only has a label)

2: Label s_i by labeling rules and get $Tag = (t_1, t_2...t_n)$
3: ES : an empty string ; $Max = |Tag|$
4: **if** $L1 \in Tag$ **then**
5:   Taking $L1$ as dividing line for multiple entities
6:   **return** E
7: **else**
8:   **for each** $i \in [1, |Tag|]$ **do**
9:     **switch** (t_i)
10:    **case** $L2$:
11:      **if** $ES! ="$ **then**
12:        **if** $t_{i-1} = L4$ **then**
13:          $E \leftarrow ES + s_i; ES ="$
14:        **else if** $t_{i-1} = L3$ or $L5$ **then**
15:          $E \leftarrow ES; ES ="$
16:        **end if**
17:        **if** $i < Max$ **then**
18:          **if** $t_{i+1} = L5$ or $L2$ or $L6$ **then**
19:            $E \leftarrow s_i$
20:          **else**
21:            $ES+ = s_i$
22:          **end if**
23:        **else**
24:          $E \leftarrow s_i$
25:        **end if**
26:      **else**
27:        **if** $i < Max$ **then**
28:          **if** $t_{i+1} = L5$ or $L2$ or $L6$ **then**
29:            $E \leftarrow s_i$
30:          **else**
31:            $ES+ = s_i$

```
31:                ES+ = s_i
32:             end if
33:          else
34:             E ← s_i
35:          end if
36:       end if
37:    case L5:
38:       if ES! =″ then
39:          E ← ES; ES =″
40:       end if
41:       if i < Max then
42:          if t_{i+1} = L5 or L2 or L6 then
43:             E ← s_i
44:          else
45:             ES+ = s_i
46:          end if
47:       else
48:          E ← s_i
49:       end if
50:    case L6:
51:       if i = Max then
52:          E ← ES + s_i
53:       else
54:          ES+ = s_i
55:       end if
56:    case L4:
57:       if i = Max then
58:          E ← ES + s_i
59:       else
60:          ES+ = s_i
61:       end if
62:    case L3:
63:       if i = Max then
64:          E ← ES + s_i
65:       else
66:          ES+ = s_i
67:       end if
68:    end switch
69:   end for
70: end if
71: return  E
```

References

1. National Health and Family Planning Commission of the People's Republic of China. Basic Specifications for Electronic Medical Records (Trial). http://www.nhc.gov.cn/zwgk/wtwj/201304/a99a0bae95be4a27a8b7d883cd0bc3aa.shtml
2. National Health and Family Planning Commission of the People's Republic of China. Medical Record Basic Specification. http://www.nhfpc.gov.cn/yzygj/s3585u/201002/0517a8235224ee0912a5d855a9d249f.shtml
3. Sun, W., Rumshisky, A., Uzuner, O.: Evaluating temporal relations in clinical text: 2012 i2b2 Challenge. J. Am. Med. Inf. Assoc. Jamia 20(5), 806–813 (2013)
4. Bethard, S., Derczynski, L., Savova, G., Pustejovsky, J., Verhagen, M.: SemEval-2015 Task 6: Clinical TempEval. In: Proceedings of the 9th International Workshop on Semantic Evaluation (SemEval 2015), pp. 806–814. Association for Computational, Denver, Colorado (2015)
5. Bethard, S., Savova, G., Chen, W.-T., Derczynski, L., Pustejovsky, J., Verhagen, M.: SemEval-2016 Task 12: Clinical TempEval. In: Proceedings of the 10th International Workshop on Semantic Evaluation (SemEval-2016), pp. 1052–1062. Association for Computational, San Diego, California (2016)
6. Bethard, S., Savova, G., Palmer, M., Pustejovsky, J.: SemEval-2017 Task 12: Clinical TempEval. In: Proceedings of the 11th International Workshop on Semantic Evaluation (SemEval-2017), pp. 565–572. Association for Computational, Vancouver, Canada (2017)
7. Ramponi, A., Goot, R., Lombardo, R., et al.: Biomedical event extraction as sequence labeling. In: The 2020 Conference on Empirical Methods in Natural Language Processing (EMNLP) 2020
8. Li, D., Huang, L., Ji, H., Han, J.: Biomedical Event Extraction based on Knowledge-driven Tree-LSTM. In: Proceedings of the 2019 Conference of the North American Chapter of the Association for Computational Linguistics, Human Language Technologies, vol. 1, pp. 1421–1430. Minneapolis, Minnesota (2019)
9. Huang, K.-H., Yang, M., Peng, N.: Biomedical event extraction with hierarchical knowledge graphs. In: Findings of the Association for Computational Linguistics: EMNLP 2020, pp. 1277–1285
10. CHIP 2018 task 1. http://icrc.hitsz.edu.cn/chip2018/Task.html
11. Han, X., et al.: overview of the ccks 2019 knowledge graph evaluation track: entity, relation, event and QA. arXiv preprint arXiv:2003.03875 (2020)
12. Li, X., Wen, Q., Lin, H., et al.: Overview of CCKS 2020 Task 3: named entity recognition and event extraction in Chinese electronic medical records. Data Intell. 3(5), 376–388 (2021)
13. CHIP 2021 task 2. http://cips-chip.org.cn/2021/eval2
14. Bin Ji, et al.: A multi neural networks based approach to complex Chinese medical named entity recognition (2019)
15. Dai, S., et al.: Few-shot medical event extraction based on pre-trained language model (2020)
16. Gan, Z., et al.: Enhance both text and label: combination strategies for improving the generalization ability of medical entity extraction. In: Qin, B., Wang, H., Liu, M., Zhang, J. (eds.) CCKS 2021 - Evaluation Track. CCKS 2021. Communications in Computer and Information Science, vol. 1553 Springer, Singapore (2022). https://doi.org/10.1007/978-981-19-0713-5_11
17. Lample, G., et al.: Neural architectures for named entity recognition. In: Proceedings of the 2016 Conference of the North American Chapter of the Association for Computational Linguistics: Human Language Technologies (2016)

18. PCL-MedBERT from Peng Cheng Lab. https://www.pcl.ac.cn/html/943/2020-08-22/content-3400.html
19. Zhong, Z., et al.: A frustratingly easy approach for entity and relation extraction. North American Chapter of the Association for Computational Linguistics Association for Computational Linguistics (2021)
20. Wang, X., Weber, L., et al.: Biomedical event extraction as multi-turn question answering. In: Proceedings of the 11th International Workshop on Health Text Mining and Information Analysis 2020, pp. 88–96
21. Bin, J., et al.: Research on Chinese medical named entity recognition based on collaborative cooperation of multiple neural network models. J. Biomed. Inform. **104**, 103395 (2020). https://doi.org/10.1016/j.jbi.2020.103395
22. Bin, Ji., et al.: A hybrid approach for named entity recognition in Chinese electronic medical record. BMC Med. Inf. Decis. Making **19** (S2), 64 (2019). https://doi.org/10.1186/s12911-019-0767-2

Infusing Dependency Syntax Information into a Transformer Model for Document-Level Relation Extraction from Biomedical Literature

Ming Yang[1], Yijia Zhang[1(✉)], Da Liu[1], Wei Du[1], Yide Di[1], and Hongfei Lin[2]

[1] School of Information Science and Technology, Dalian Maritime University,
Dalian 116024, Liaoning, China
zhangyijia@dlmu.edu.cn
[2] School of Computer Science and Technology, Dalian University of Technology,
Dalian 116023, Lioaoning, China

Abstract. In biomedical domain, document-level relation extraction is a challenging task that offers a new and more effective approach for long and complex text mining. Studies have shown that the Transformer models the dependencies of any two tokens without regard to their syntax-level dependency in the sequence. In this work, we propose a **D**ependency **S**yntax **T**ransformer **M**odel, i.e., the DSTM model, to improve the Transformer's ability in long-range modeling dependencies. Three methods are proposed for introducing dependency syntax information into the Transformer to enhance the attention of tokens with dependencies in a sentence. The dependency syntax Transformer model improves the Transformer's ability to handle long text in document-level relation extraction. Our experimental results on the document-level relation extraction dataset CDR in the biomedical field prove the validity of the DSTM model, and the experimental results on the generic domain dataset DocRED prove the universality.

Keywords: Document-level relation extraction · Dependency syntax information · Transformer model · Attention mechanism · Biomedical literature

1 Introduction

Relation extraction extracts unknown relational facts from plain text, which is a significant step to enable further text mining. Automatic extraction of biomedical information has attracted much attention from researchers in recent years. Previously relation extraction focused on intra-sentence relation extraction [1,2]. However, many facts not only exist in a single sentence but are also distributed in multiple sentences. Several studies [3,4] have shown that more than 30%–40% of relational facts exist in multiple sentences. Therefore, relation extraction has extended to the document level.

© The Author(s), under exclusive license to Springer Nature Singapore Pte Ltd. 2023
B. Tang et al. (Eds.): CHIP 2022, CCIS 1772, pp. 37–52, 2023.
https://doi.org/10.1007/978-981-19-9865-2_3

The document-level relation extraction task has many challenges. Document-level relation extraction has a broader scope of action, longer texts and a more dispersed distribution of information than sentence-level relation extraction. A document contains multiple entity pairs. One entity pair can occur many times in the document associated with distinct relations for document-level relation extraction, in contrast to one relation per entity pair for sentence-level relation extraction. For example, Fig. 1 shows an instance of CDR. There is a relation of 'CID' between etomidate and pain, swelling, nausea and so on. We must correctly analyze the relation between entity etomidate and every other sentence to get the answer. The analysis of the CID relation between entities etomidate and nausea mainly span the entire article. This requires that the document-level relation extraction model has an excellent ability to model long and complex text dependencies.

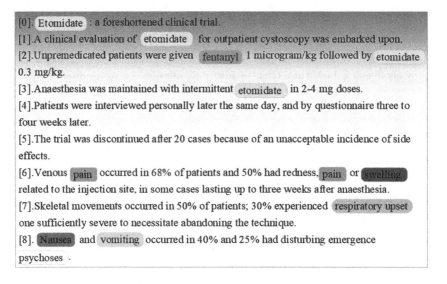

Fig. 1. An example from the CDR dataset.

Document-level relation extraction has developed rapidly over the past two years [5–7]. The transformer-based pretraining model has enormously contributed to natural language processing (NLP). However, Transformer-based pretraining models model dependencies for any two tokens without regard to their syntax-level dependency in the sequences. This prevents the Transformer from modeling dependencies of sentences in long-range and reasoning relation between entities.

It has been proved effective to use dependency syntax trees of input sentences in relation extraction to capture long-range syntactic features that are difficult to obtain only from surface forms. In recent years, dependency syntax information has been introduced into the design of graph structures to model the dependencies between entities. Most studies combined a dependency syntax graph with Graph Convolutional Network (GCN) [8] and its variants for feature extraction of sentences and then interactively learned with BERT [9]. But this approach separates the feature construction process so that BERT cannot really benefit from the dependency syntax information due to the heterogeneity of BERT and GCN.

In this paper, we propose a DSTM model, i.e., a dependency syntax information-guided Transformer model, to enhance the Transformer model's ability to model the dependencies between tokens in long-range text in document-level relation extraction. First, we use a dependency syntax parser to parse the dependencies between tokens and design a document-level dependency syntax tree. Then three alternative transformations, direct transformation, biaffine transformation and decomposed linear transformation, are proposed to integrate dependency syntax information into the Transformer model. Finally, the optimal transformation method is chosen based on the model characteristics and data distribution to introduce the dependency syntax information into the Transformer. The dependency syntax information runs through the whole process of the Transformer. We conduct comprehensive experiments on two datasets, DocRED and CDR, to demonstrate the effectiveness of the proposed approach. Our research contributions can be summarized as follows:

- We propose a DSTM model, a Transformer model guided by dependency syntax information in alternative ways, for document-level relation extraction tasks. The DSTM model has improved Transformer's ability to model long texts dependencies by enhancing attention between two tokens with dependencies in a sentence.
- A dependency syntax tree is built at the document level, and three different alternative fusion methods are designed to fuse the dependency syntax information into the Transformer. The best method is selected according to the model characteristics and data distribution.
- We conduct experiments on the DSTM model on two open datasets and perform a comparative analysis of the experimental results. The experimental results demonstrate that the DSTM model enhances the Transformer's ability in long-range modeling text and promotes the Transformer for document-level tasks.

2 Method

The overall structure of our proposed model is shown in Fig. 2, where the right half of Fig. 2 is the detailed structure of the DSTM model. The primary process is rough as follows: First, the text is put into the DSTM model to generate the high-quality contextual representation of each token. Second, the feature representation of the entity is constructed. Then, the entity features are connected with the distance features between the entities to enrich the entity features further. Finally, the entity features are fed to the sigmoid function to extract relations.

2.1   Document-Level Dependency Syntax Tree

Dependency syntax analysis is performed on each sentence processed by tokenization to obtain the corresponding dependency syntax tree. In this paper, we use Stanford CoreNLP[1] to parse the dependency syntax information of each sentence. Each dependency syntax tree has only a root node that does not depend on any other token in the sentence. Subsequently, the root node of the latter sentence is linked to the root node of the previous sentence. Make the root node of the subsequent sentence dependent on the root node of the previous sentence to enhance the degree of association between the two sentences. By repeating the above, a dependency syntax tree is generated for the entire document to represent the dependencies between tokens throughout the document. For example, the article's document-level dependency syntax tree structure in Fig. 1 is detailed in Part 2 of Fig. 4. This dependent syntax tree can indicate the dependencies of Mawene and Mozambique entities. Finally, the dependency syntax tree is transformed into the corresponding adjacency matrix A.

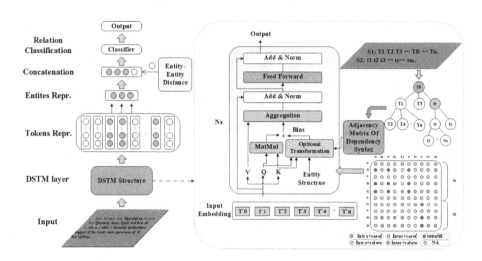

Fig. 2. Complete schematic view of our proposed model.

2.2   DSTM for Document-Level Relation Extraction

Given a token sequence $x = (x_1, x_2, x_3, ..., x_n)$ as input. First, we obtain the embedding of each token from a BERT embedding. The overall framework of BERT comprises several layers of transformer encoder. Each layer of the encoder comprises a layer of multihead attention and a layer of feedforward attention. In

---

[1] https://stanfordnlp.github.io/CoreNLP/.

the l_{th} layer, the token embedding $x_i^l \in R^{d_{in}}$ is mapped to the query, key and value vectors, respectively:

$$q_i^l = x_i^l W_i^Q, k_i^l = x_i^l W_i^K, v_i^l = x_i^l W_i^V \tag{1}$$

where $W_i^Q, W_i^K, W_i^V \in R^{d_{in} \times d_{out}}$. We calculate the attention score between any two tokens using vectors q and k in the self-attention mechanism. The unstructured attention score is as follows:

$$e_{ij}^l = \frac{q_i^l k_j^{l^T}}{\sqrt{d}} \tag{2}$$

Dependency syntax information represents the interdependence between tokens. Therefore, attention between two tokens with a dependency should be more critical than attention between any other two tokens. The dependency syntax information enhances the weight between two tokens with a dependency syntax relation. Firstly, the attention bias, i.e., the parameter Bias, generated by the adjacency matrix of the dependency syntax tree guides q and k. Next, an unstructured attention score and attention bias are integrated into the final attention score, as detailed in the right half of Fig. 2.

$$\hat{e}_{ij}^l = e_{ij}^l + Bias(q_i^l, k_j^l, A_{ij}) \tag{3}$$

where $\hat{e}_{ij}^l$ is the attention score guided by the dependent syntax information.

How do we get Bias? We propose three alternative calculation methods to incorporate the dependency syntax structure A_{ij} into the Transformer structure: direct transformation, biaffine transformation and decom transformation. The detailed process of the three transformations is as follows:

Direct Transformation:
After obtaining the attention scores via q and k, the direct transformation module directly enacts the dependency syntax matrix on the attention scores. Only the attention value between the two tokens with dependency syntax relations is retained in this method and is regarded as the final attention bias:

$$Bias(q_i^l, k_j^l, A_{ij}) = (q_i^l k_j^{l^T}) * A_{ij} + b_{l,A_{ij}} \tag{4}$$

where A_{ij} is 1 if x_i depends on x_j. Otherwise, A_{ij} is 0. $b_{l,A_{ij}}$ is the prior bias that we model for the dependencies of each independent context.

Biaffine Transformation:
The Biaffine Transformation computes the bias as:

$$Bias(q_i^l, k_j^l, A_{ij}) = (q_i^l W_{bili} k_j^{l^T}) * A_{ij} + b_{l,A_{ij}} \tag{5}$$

where $W_{bili} \in R^{d_{in} \times d_{out}}$ is parameterized the adjacency matrix of the dependency syntax information A_{ij} as a trainable neural network layer, which simultaneously and directionally processes the query and key vector and projects them into a single-dimensional deviation.

Decomposed Linear Transformation:

For decomposed linear transformation, inspired by [10] how decomposed the word embedding and position embedding in Transformer, we introduce a bias for the query and key vectors, respectively:

$$Bias(q_i^l, k_j^l, A_{ij}) = (q_i^l K_l^T + Q_l k_j^{l~T}) * A_{ij} + b_{l,A_{ij}} \tag{6}$$

where $K_l, Q_l \in R^{d_{in} \times d_{out}}$ are also trainable neural layers.

The Optional Transformation module regulates the attention flow from x_i to x_j. The dependency syntax information runs through the entire model. Furthermore, we also introduced the entity structure in SSAN [11] into Transformer via biaffine. We softmax $\hat{e}_{ij}^l$ and aggregate it with the value vector:

$$x_i^{l+1} = \sum_{j=1}^{n} \frac{\exp \hat{e}_{ij}^l}{\sum_{k=1}^{n} \exp \hat{e}_{ij}^l} v_j^l \tag{7}$$

where $x_i^{l+1} \in R^{d_{out}}$ is the updated contextual representation of x_i^l.

Additionally, we construct the distance feature $D = (d_1, d_2, d_3, ..., d_n) \in R^{d_d \times d_d}$ between entities, and the distance between the i_{th} and the j_{th} entities are represented as d_{ij}. The constructed entity representation $e_i^{'}$ is connected with the distance feature between entities d_{ij} to form the final entity representation e_i. We obtain a comprehensive and rich context representation of each token.

$$e_i = e_i^{'} \oplus d_{ij} \tag{8}$$

We calculate the relation probability of each entity pair in the case that the relation is r, using a bilinear function:

$$P_r(e_s, e_o) = sigmoid(e_s W_r e_o) \tag{9}$$

where $W_r \in R^{d_e \times d_e}$, r stands for relation type. The DSTM model is trained using cross-entropy loss:

$$L = \sum_{<s,o>} \sum_{r} CrossEntropy(P_r(e_s, e_o), \overline{y}_r(e_s, e_o)) \tag{10}$$

where $\overline{y}_r$ is the target label.

3   Experiments

3.1   Datasets

We evaluate our DSTM model on two datasets, the document-level biomedical relation extraction dataset CDR and the public document-level relation extraction dataset DocRED.

CDR. The Chemical-Disease Relations dataset is a biomedical dataset constructed using PubMed abstracts. It contains 1500 human-annotated documents

Table 1. The details of the CDR dataset.

Datasets	Number of documents	Chemical type	Disease type	CID relation
Train	500	1476	1965	1038
Dev	500	1507	1865	1012
Test	500	1435	1988	1066

Table 2. The details of the DocRED dataset.

Datasets	Number of documents	Relation type	Instances	Fact
Train	3053	96	38262	34715
Dev	1000	96	12332	11790
Test	1000	96	12842	12101

Note: Number of documents, relation type, instances and fact denote the number of articles, the number of relations, the number of relation instances and the number of relational facts in the training set, the dev set and the test set, respectively.

with 4409 annotated chemicals, 5818 diseases, and 3116 chemical-disease inter-actions. CDR is a binary classification task that aims at identifying induced relation from chemical entity to disease entity. The details of the datasets are shown in Table 1.

DocRED. The DocRED dataset is a large-scale document-level information extraction dataset generated by combining articles from Wikipedia and Wiki-data. The DocRED dataset covers 132375 entities and 96 frequent relation types. There are 97 target relations in this article, including None. More than 40.7% of the relational facts in the DocRED should be considered in multiple sentences to predict the relations. The details of the datasets are shown in Table 2.

3.2 Experimental Setting

Some essential hyperparameters are listed in Table 4. It is worth noting that the BERT base and SciBERT are used in the DSTM model for the CDR, and RoBERTa is used for DocRED. Following the SSAN model work, we use Ign F1 and F1 measures as evaluation metrics for the document-level relation extraction performance, where Ign F1 denotes the F1 scores excluding the relational facts shared by the training, dev and test sets.

3.3 CDR Results

Table 3 illustrates the comprehensive experimental results of the DSTM model in detail on the CDR dataset, which outperform other models in previous work. We also conduct a comprehensive comparative analysis of these models from different perspectives.

Table 3. Comparison results on CDR.

Model	Dev F1	Test F1	Intra-F1/Inter-F1
BRAN (2018) [12]	–	62.1	–/–
EoG (2019) [5]	63.6	63.6	68.2/50.9
LSR (2020) [6]	–	61.2	66.2/50.3
LSR w/o MDP (2020) [6]	–	64.8	68.9/53.1
SSAN$_{Biaffine}$-BERT_Base (2021) [11]	60.56	60.65	67.73/46.13
SSAN$_{Biaffine}$-SciBERT (2021) [11]	67.43	64.66	71.45/50.4
BERT_Base	61.45	60.28	67.65/45.2
SciBERT	66.01	65.06	70.77/52.87
DSTM$_{Direct}$-SciBERT	67.54	63.96	70.17/51.13
DSTM$_{Biaffine}$-SciBERT	66.93	66.36	72.27/53.49
DSTM$_{Decomp}$-SciBERT	67.96	**67.23**	**72.86/54.86**
DSTM$_{Direct}$-RoBERTa_Base	52.5	51.9	58.53/32.07
DSTM$_{Biaffine}$-RoBERTa_Base	65.37	64.9	70.14/50.4
DSTM$_{Decomp}$-RoBERTa_Base	61.88	61.32	68.24/48.56

Notes: 'Intra-F1' denotes the F1 of intra-sentence relation, 'Inter-F1' indicates the F1 of inter-sentence relation.

EOG and LSR are based on the graph structure for structural reasoning. The graph structure is generally used after BiLSTM or BERT. However, the differences in the nature and structure of the sequence and graph structure seriously affect task research. On the CDR dataset, we not only used BERT to process texts but also took advantage of the superiority of SciBERT in processing biomedical texts. The SSAN model defines six entity structures to guide the flow of attention in BERT. It can be observed that the DSTM$_{Biaffine}$-SciBERT model increases Intra-F1 and Inter-F1 by 0.82 and 3.09 compared with SSAN on the test set. This shows that the DSTM model is more advantageous in dealing with inter-sentence relations. In addition, RoBERTa was also used for the CDR dataset, but the results were not satisfactory. The experimental results show that SciBERT is more suitable for NLP tasks in the biomedical domain. In general, the experimental results indicate that the Transformer based on dependent syntax

Table 4. Hyperparamters setting.

Pretraining model	BERT base/RoBERTa base	SciBERT
Hyperparamters	Value	Value
Batch size	4	4
Learning rate	5e−5	2e−5
Epoch	40	40
Max_ent_cnt	42	42
Seed	42	42

Table 5. Comparison results on DocRED.

Model	Dev	Test
	F1	Ign F1/F1
ContexAware (2019) [3]	51.09	48.40/50.70
EoG (2019) [5]	52.15	49.48/51.82
BERT Two-Phase (2019a) [13]	54.42	−/53.92
GloVe+LSR (2020) [6]	55.17	52.15/54.18
BERT+LSR (2020) [6]	59.00	56.97/59.05
HINBERT (2020) [14]	56.31	53.70/55.60
CorefBERT Base (2020) [15]	57.51	54.54/56.96
CorefRoBERTa (2020) [15]	59.93	57.68/59.91
DISCO-RE (2021) [7]	57.78	55.01/55.70
SSAN$_{\text{Biaffine}}$-BERT_Base (2021) [11]	58.48	55.50/57.69
SSAN$_{\text{Biaffine}}$-RoBERTa_Base (2021) [11]	60.89	57.71/59.94
BERT_Base	58.60	55.08/57.54
RoBERTa_Base	59.52	57.27/59.48
DSTM$_{\text{Biaffine}}$-BERT_Base	58.84	56.03/58.19
DSTM$_{\text{Direct}}$-RoBERTa_Base	57.30	54.84/57.27
DSTM$_{\text{Biaffine}}$-RoBERTa_Base	60.44	**58.53/60.67**
DSTM$_{\text{Decomp}}$-RoBERTa_Base	60.23	57.69/59.89
DSTM$_{\text{Biaffine}}$-SciBERT	55.20	53.71/55.68

Note: Test results are obtained by submitting to the official Codalab.

information, i.e., the DSTM model, is excellent for the document-level biomedical relation extraction task.

The different performances of the three alternative transformation modes are also apparent in Table 3. Surprisingly, the direct transformation approach does not bring superior effects to the model. We suspect this is because the adjacency matrix of the dependency syntax information is a discrete structure, and direct import does not bring broad auxiliary effects to the end-to-end model. The result of the decomposed linear transformation is slightly better than biaffine transformation, which is the best way to introduce dependency syntax information into SciBERT. In summary, the experimental results show that the dependency syntax information is used to guide the Transformer-based pretraining model and is beneficial for the model to learn richer contextual information, thus facilitating progress in the document-level relation extraction task.

3.4   DocRED Results

Table 5 illustrates the comprehensive experimental results in detail on the DocRED dataset. DISCO-RE introduces rhetorical structure theory as external knowledge based on BERT. The Ign F1 and F1 of our DSTM$_{\text{Biaffine}}$ model built upon BERT are 1.02 and 2.49 higher than DISCO-RE on the test set. It can be

Table 6. Ablation study of the DSTM model on CDR.

Model	Test F1	Inter-F1/Intra-F1
DSTM$_{\text{Decomp}}$_SciBERT	67.23	54.86/72.86
- dependency_information $[(q_i^l K_l^T + Q_l k_j^{l\,T}) * A_{ij} + b_{l,A_{ij}}]$	65.46	50.85/72.35
- entity_structure	64.74	51.52/71.04

Notes: Intra-F1 denotes the F1 of intra-sentence, and inter-F1 denotes the F1 of inter-sentence.

Table 7. Ablation study of the DSTM model on DocRED.

Model	Dev F1	Ign F1/F1
DSTM$_{\text{Biaffine}}$_RoBERTa_Base	60.44	58.53/60.67
- dependency_information $[(q_i^l W_{bili} k_j^{l\,T}) * A_{ij} + b_{l,A_{ij}}]$	59.52	57.27/59.94
- entity_structure	59.87	57.22/59.43
- entity_inf	60.24	57.26/59.48

Notes: Ign F1 denotes Ign F1 in the test set. '-' indicates removing the corresponding component. 'entity_inf' denotes type, position and distance between entities.

observed that the DSTM$_{\text{Biaffine}}$_RoBERTa_Base model increases Ign F1 and F1 by 0.82 and 0.73 compared with SSAN on the test set. DSTM$_{\text{Biaffine}}$_RoBERTa model performs best in the DocRED dataset. The different distribution of datasets results in different performances of fusion methods. We also tried SciBERT for the DocRED dataset, but the result was disappointing. In general, the experimental results on DocRED indicate the DSTM has strong applicability and universality.

3.5   Ablation Study

In this section, we conduct ablation experiments on CDR and DocRED datasets to explore the contribution of each component to the overall performance. As shown in Table 6, we first explore the impact caused by dependency syntax information for the overall model. When dependency syntax information is removed from the DSTM, the F1 drops 1.77. This experimental result demonstrates that dependency syntax information is critical in obtaining superior performance. Next, we evaluated the impact of entity structure and other entity information for the overall model. The F1 results all show varying degrees of decline. The ablation experiments of the DocRED dataset are shown in Table 7. Overall, these experimental results show that each dependency plays an essential role when applying the DSTM model to document-level relation extraction.

We also conduct a comparative experiment on the number of RoBERTa layers with dependency syntax information on the DocRED dataset. First, we select the different layers of RoBERTa with dependency syntax information from front to back to obtain the corresponding DSTM model. Then, we apply it to the

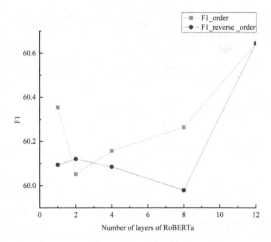

Fig. 3. Effect of the number of layers in RoBERTa where dependent information is present on DocRED dataset.

document-level relation extraction task to obtain the result as an F1_order. Similarly, an F1_reverse_order is obtained by selecting the number of layers of RoBERTa from back to front. Comparing the two results in Fig. 3 shows that the performance improvement is significant when the dependency syntax information is only present in the first layer but not so much when it is only present in the eleventh layer. These experimental results indicate that the dependency syntax information plays a more significant role at the bottom layer of RoBERTa than at the top layer. The main reason is that the dependency syntax information is derived from analyzing the sentence's syntactic structure, and the tokens information at the bottom of RoBERTa is closer to the tokens information of the original sentence. This result is in line with our expectations. Nevertheless, the dependency syntax information-guided model becomes more effective as the total number of layers of RoBERTa increases.

3.6   Case Study

We selected one of the articles from the CDR dataset for detailed analysis in Fig. 4. There are 8 entities in this article and almost all CID relations require cross-sentence inference. The red of Part 4 are the relational triplet that was not correctly predicted by the SSAN model but was correctly predicted by DSTM. The baseline model implicates the relation between etomidate and pain. In addition, the baseline model assumes that fentanyl and pain, swelling, etc., have CID relations, but they do not constitute CID relations in this article. The baseline model formed a misjudgment, whereas the DSTM model correctly judged the relation. It follows that the document-level dependency syntax tree was

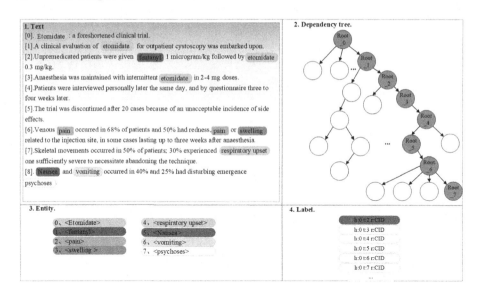

Fig. 4. An example of the document-level dependency syntax tree and its corresponding document, entities and labels of CDR dataset.

applied to the Transformer-based pretraining model to alleviate the problem of document-level tasks on long texts, proving the validity of our innovative ideas.

This paper visualizes the attention values between the entities in the article based on the SSAN and DSTM models, respectively. As shown in Fig. 5, the attention values of the entities etomidate and pain, swelling, nausea, and vomiting are significantly higher on the DSTM model than on the SSAN. This phenomenon highlights the role of dependent syntax information in guiding the Transformer-based pretraining model in terms of attention. Although the attention between entities fentanyl and pain, swelling, respiratory upset, nausea and vomiting are similar on the DSTM and the SSAN. However, the combined evaluation of attention on the DSTM model is still lower than that on SSAN. This phenomenon is still advantageous to our task.

Finally, although the DSTM model is compatible with the pretraining model, there is still a distributed gap between the newly introduced and originally trained parameters, which hinders the performance of the DSTM model to a certain extent. The SSAN model gives us a new perspective to address this problem. The model is tested after training a distantly supervised dataset in DocRED. In future work, we will use this method to enhance the capabilities of the DSTM model for document-level relation extraction tasks, and we anticipate promising results. In general, the DSTM model remains competitive for document-level relation extraction.

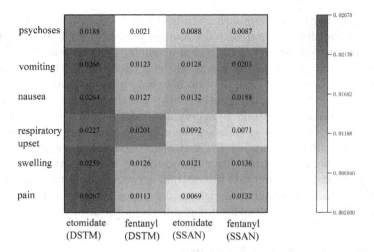

Fig. 5. Examples of the attention value between some entities.

4   Related Work

4.1   Document-Level Relation Extraction

Document-level relation extraction is more challenging than sentence-level relation extraction. Strategies based on the design of feature extractors at different levels attempt to extract hierarchical features at the token, sentence, and document levels through networks at different levels. It concatenates the features at different levels to classify the relations between entities. A typical example is that [14] uses Bi-directional Long Short-Term Memory (BiLSTM) to extract feature sequences at different levels. It uses the attention mechanism to obtain the overall feature weighted to obtain the local and global information of the entity. This category has challenges dealing with entity relations in long texts or across sentences.

The global graph-based approach uses GCN [16,17] or GAT [18] to iterate the designed graph and then obtain the structural features of each node after smoothing. Some papers proposed using multiple hierarchical graph neural networks to extract structural features at different levels, considering that a single global graph may not be able to obtain complete global information. For example, GAIN [19] constructed two graphs at the mentioned and entity levels. After obtaining better mention embeddings via the mention-level GCN, it will receive more meaningful entity embeddings. DHG [20] constructed words and sentences into the first graph to mine the structural features of the entity and constructed relation reasoning subgraphs of mentions and entities to obtain information on the reasoning level.

The BERT hardcoded approach attempts to model the global confidence with the original transformer, and BERT is not only an encoder but also a feature extractor in relation extraction tasks. For example, [21] introduced the labels of entity classes and global entities based on the original BERT. BiLinear outputs the category information of the relation between entity pairs and implements a one pass model. In paper [22], mention-entity matching, relation detection and relation fact alignment subtasks were designed in BERT for document-level relation extraction. SSAN [11] establishes the corresponding entity structure information by determining whether the two mentioned entities were in the same sentence and refer to the same entity, introducing it into the attention score calculation part, and finally outputs the relation between the entity pairs. However, Transformer-based pretraining models model dependencies for any two tokens without regard to their syntax-level dependency in the sequences.

4.2   Dependency Syntax Structure

Dependency trees of input sentences are used in models and have proven to be effective in relation extraction. Traditional statistical models handle dependency information by combining different lexical, syntactic and semantic features [23]. However, sparse features and reliance on features created by external systems pose a significant challenge to the model processing task. Recent research has focused on document-level dependency graphs for encoding through dependent syntactic information combined with GCNs to capture useful long-range syntactic information [24]. Recently, Transformer models have shown excellent performance in NLP. However, Transformer structure model dependencies for any two tokens without regard to their syntax-level dependency in the sequences. To solve this problem, we design the DSTM model.

5   Conclusion and Future Work

In this work, we propose the DSTM model for document-level relation extraction. We designed a document-level dependency syntax tree and proposed three fusion approaches. The best approach was chosen to incorporate the dependency syntax information into the Transformer to enhance the ability of the Transformer to model long-range dependencies. The results obtained on CDR demonstrate the superiority of the DSTM model for document-level biomedical relation extraction, and the results on DocRED demonstrate the applicability of the DSTM model.

There is still some room to improve with future work. One possible improvement is to construct document-level dependency syntax trees to display the dependency relations between tokens better. A second possibility is finding a way to solve the entity overlap problem in relation extraction.

Acknowledgements. This work is supported by grant from the Natural Science Foundation of China (No. 62072070).

References

1. Zhang, T., Leng, J., Liu, Y.: Deep learning for drug-drug interaction extraction from the literature: a review. Briefings Bioinform. **21**(5), 1609–1627 (2020). https://doi.org/10.1093/bib/bbz087
2. Li, Z., Sun, Y., Zhu, J., Tang, S., Zhang, C., Ma, H.: Improve relation extraction with dual attention-guided graph convolutional networks. Neural Comput. Appl. **33**(6), 1773–1784 (2020). https://doi.org/10.1007/s00521-020-05087-z
3. Yao, Y., et al.: Docred: a large-scale document-level relation extraction dataset. In: Proceedings of the 57th Annual Meeting of the Association for Computational Linguistics, pp. 764–777 (2019). https://doi.org/10.18653/v1/P19-1074
4. Jin, L., Song, L., Zhang, Y., Xu, K., Ma, W., Yu, D.: Relation extraction exploiting full dependency forests. In: Proceedings of the AAAI Conference on Artificial Intelligence, vol. 34, n. 05, pp. 8034–8041 (2020). https://doi.org/10.1609/aaai.v34i05.6313
5. Christopoulou, F., Miwa, M., Ananiadou, S.: Connecting the dots: document-level neural relation extraction with edge-oriented graphs. In: Proceedings of the 2019 Conference on Empirical Methods in Natural Language Processing and the 9th International Joint Conference on Natural Language Processing (EMNLP-IJCNLP), pp. 4925–4936 (2019). https://doi.org/10.18653/v1/D19-1498
6. Nan, G., Guo, Z., Sekulić, I., Lu, W.: Reasoning with latent structure refinement for document-level relation extraction. In: Proceedings of the 58th Annual Meeting of the Association for Computational Linguistics, pp. 1546–1557 (2020). https://doi.org/10.18653/v1/2020.acl-main.141
7. Wang, H., Qin, K., Lu, G., Yin, J., Zakari, R.Y., Owusu, J.W.: Document-level relation extraction using evidence reasoning on RST-graph. Knowl.-Based Syst. **228**, 107274 (2021). https://doi.org/10.1016/j.knosys.2021.107274
8. Kipf, T.N., Welling, M.: Semi-supervised classification with graph convolutional networks. In: 5th International Conference on Learning Representations (ICLR) (2017)
9. Tang, H., Ji, D., Li, C., Zhou, Q.: Dependency graph enhanced dual-transformer structure for aspect-based sentiment classification. In: Proceedings of the 58th Annual Meeting of the Association for Computational Linguistics, pp. 6578–6588 (2020). https://doi.org/10.18653/v1/2020.acl-main.588
10. Dai, Z., Yang, Z., Yang, Y., Carbonell, J., Le, Q.V., Salakhutdinov, R.: Transformer-xl: attentive language models beyond a fixed-length context. In: Proceedings of the 57th Conference of the Association for Computational Linguistics (ACL) (Long Papers), vol. 1, pp. 2978–2988 (2019). https://doi.org/10.18653/v1/p19-1285
11. Xu, B., Wang, Q., Lyu, Y., Zhu, Y., Mao, Z.: Entity structure within and throughout: modeling mention dependencies for document-level relation extraction. In: Proceedings of the AAAI Conference on Artificial Intelligence, vol. 35, no. 16, pp. 14149–14157 (2021)
12. Verga, P., Strubell, E., Mccallum, A.: Simultaneously self-attending to all mentions for full-abstract biological relation extraction. In: Proceedings of the 2018 Conference of the North American Chapter of the Association for Computational Linguistics: Human Language Technologies, NAACL-HLT, Volume 1 (Long Papers), pp. 872–884 (2018). https://doi.org/10.18653/v1/n18-1080
13. Wang, H., Focke, C., Sylvester, R., Mishra, N., Wang, W.: Fine-tune BERT for DOCRED with two-step process. arXiv preprint arXiv:1909.11898 (2019)

14. Tang, H., et al.: HIN: hierarchical inference network for document-level relation extraction. Adv. Knowl. Discov. Data Min. **12084**, 197 (2020). https://doi.org/10.1007/978-3-030-47426-3_16

15. Ye, D., et al.: Coreferential reasoning learning for language representation. In: Proceedings of the 2020 Conference on Empirical Methods in Natural Language Processing (EMNLP), pp. 7170–7186 (2020). https://doi.org/10.18653/v1/2020.emnlp-main.582

16. Quirk, C., Poon, H.: Distant supervision for relation extraction beyond the sentence boundary. In: Proceedings of the 15th Conference of the European Chapter of the Association for Computational Linguistics: (Volume 1: Long Papers), pp. 1171–1182 (2016). https://doi.org/10.18653/v1/E17-1110

17. Sahu, S.K., Christopoulou, F., Miwa, M., Ananiadou, S.: Inter-sentence relation extraction with document-level graph convolutional neural network. In: Proceedings of the 57th Annual Meeting of the Association for Computational Linguistics, pp. 4309–4316 (2019). https://doi.org/10.18653/v1/P19-1423

18. Xu, W., Chen, K., Zhao, T.: Document-level relation extraction with reconstruction. In: The 35th AAAI Conference on Artificial Intelligence (AAAI-21), pp. 14167–14175 (2021)

19. Zeng, S., Xu, R., Chang, B., Li, L.: Double graph based reasoning for document-level relation extraction. In: Proceedings of the 2020 Conference on Empirical Methods in Natural Language Processing (EMNLP), pp. 1630–1640 (2020). https://doi.org/10.18653/v1/2020.emnlp-main.127

20. Zhang, Z., et al.: Document-level relation extraction with dual-tier heterogeneous graph. In: Proceedings of the 28th International Conference on Computational Linguistics, pp. 1630–1641 (2020). https://doi.org/10.18653/v1/2020.coling-main.143

21. Han, X., Wang, L.: A novel document-level relation extraction method based on BERT and entity information. IEEE Access **8**, 96912–96919 (2020). https://doi.org/10.1109/ACCESS.2020.2996642

22. Xiao, C., et al.: Denoising relation extraction from document-level distant supervision. In: Proceedings of the 2020 Conference on Empirical Methods in Natural Language Processing (EMNLP), pp. 3683–3688 (2020). https://doi.org/10.18653/v1/2020.emnlp-main.300

23. Kambhatla, N.: Combining lexical, syntactic, and semantic features with maximum entropy models for information extraction. In: Proceedings of the ACL Interactive Poster and Demonstration Sessions, pp. 178–181 (2004)

24. Nan, G., Guo, Z., Sekulic, I., Lu, W.: Reasoning with latent structure refinement for document-level relation extraction. In: ACL 2020, Online, 5–10 July 2020, pp. 1546–1557 (2020). https://doi.org/10.18653/v1/2020.acl-main.141

A Review of Biomedical Event Trigger Word Detection

Xueyan Zhang[1], Xinyu He[1,2,3(✉)], Siyu Liu[1], and Yonggong Ren[1(✉)]

[1] School of Computer and Technology, Liaoning Normal University, Dalian, China
hexinyu@lnnu.edu.cn, 444801898@qq.com
[2] Information and Communication Engineering Postdoctoral Research Station, Dalian
University of Technology, Dalian, China
[3] Postdoctoral Workstation of Dalian Yongjia Electronic Technology Co., Ltd., Dalian, China

Abstract. Trigger words refer to the characteristic words that can reveal the nature of the event, marking the occurrence of the event. Trigger word recognition is one of the sub-tasks of event extraction, which is an important part of information extraction. In recent years, with the continuous development of natural language processing in biomedical field, many scholars have developed various trigger word recognition methods. In this paper, we firstly introduce the background, concept, goal and significance of the trigger word detection, then classify the trigger word recognition methods, elaborate on advantages, disadvantages and applicable conditions of dictionary-based, rule-based, machine learning-based, deep learning-based methods and some hybrid models. Finally, we analysis the problems and challenges of biomedical event trigger word detection, and look forward to the future research direction.

Keywords: Biomedical event · Event extraction · Trigger word recognition ·
Deep learning

1 Introduction

In the current era of medical big data, people pay more and more attention to medical health and explore the treatment of life health and diseases actively. With the development of information technology, the amount of biomedical data is increasing exponentially. Massive literature and resources on numerous social media platforms are of extremely high value. How to extract accurate and useful information quickly and conveniently is a crucial problem. Automated biomedical information extraction technology emerges as the times require. Biomedical information extraction usually extracts structured information from semi-structured and unstructured texts. Information extraction in the biomedical field mainly includes entity disambiguation, named entity recognition, relation extraction and event extraction [1].

Biomedical events are the fundamental units of knowledge. The significance of medical event extraction lies in driving the continuous development of automatic question and

---

X. Zhang and X. He—Contributed equally to this work.

© The Author(s), under exclusive license to Springer Nature Singapore Pte Ltd. 2023
B. Tang et al. (Eds.): CHIP 2022, CCIS 1772, pp. 53–66, 2023.
https://doi.org/10.1007/978-981-19-9865-2_4

answer, semantic search [2], disease mechanism, clinical diagnosis, drug research and development, biomedical database development, path planning [3] and so on, reducing the cost of manual marking, improving the update speed of data, and facilitating reading and mining the value of medical information.

Biomedical event extraction automatically extracts unstructured and semi-structured detailed event information from text and presents it in a structured form. It aims to identify event trigger words and the related arguments, and extract the multiple semantic relationships among fine-grained biological entities. Biomedical event extraction includes trigger word detection, argument detection, and post-processing [4].

Event trigger is the most important part of an event, which represents the occurrence of the event [5]. Event triggers usually exist in the form of verbs, verbal phrases and gerunds. In the field of biomedicine, event type refers to the description of the behavior of entities such as proteins and genes, and events are classified according to their functions. The type of trigger word directly determines the type of event. Trigger detection includes two parts: trigger identification and classification, which aims to identify biomedical trigger words in the text and classify their types. The errors of trigger word recognition affect the judgment of event type and the argument detection, which further affects the performance of the whole event detection. In summary, trigger word detection is the most important prerequisite step of biomedical event extraction.

In recent years, many scholars have proposed a variety of trigger word detection methods, however, there is a lack of systematic and in-depth combing and summary work, and the review in this direction is few. Therefore, in this paper, we summarize and classify the trigger word detection methods, elaborate the advantages, disadvantages and application of four types of methods and some hybrid models, finally analyze the problems and challenges, and look forward to the future research directions. We hope this paper can help readers to have a more comprehensive understanding of the research progress of trigger word recognition, so as to facilitate the development of future research and application work.

2   Methods of Trigger Word Recognition

2.1   Dictionary-Based Approaches

The dictionary-based methods mainly construct the trigger word dictionary by domain experts according to their professional knowledge and corpus. If the candidate word is in the trigger word dictionary, it is judged as trigger word, and vice versa.

Buyko et al. [6] constructed a dictionary from the original biomedical event corpus, selected all trigger words in the sentence manually, matched them with the corpus, and constructed a basically complete trigger word dictionary by filtering, finally the F1 value on the BioNLP09 data set was only 46.66%. Bronstein et al. [7] took some known trigger words as seeds, and expanded their trigger word dictionary through information retrieval methods.

The dictionary-based method is simple, it makes full use of context information to deal with the diversity of languages in biomedical samples, which is mainly used in early trigger word detection. However, these methods rely on manual trigger word dictionary too much, which have high labor cost, time consumption, poor portability, low generalization ability, and are not accurate and standard enough to judge the trigger word types of polysemous words accurately.

2.2 Rule-Based Approaches

The rule-based methods use strategies such as pattern matching and regular expressions to define rules [8], and then use these artificially designed rules to capture the characteristics of event triggers and their context information. If the word matches a rule in the rule template, it is judged as a trigger word; conversely, if the word does not match any of the rules in the rule template, the word is judged as a non-trigger word. Minh et al. [9] firstly selected candidate trigger words from the training set with the rule of "near proteins and with appropriate part-of-speech tagging", and then classified candidate trigger words according to the relationship between trigger words and their corresponding types in the dictionary. For the ambiguous categories, the one with the highest frequency shall prevail. Kilicoglu et al. [10] constructed rules based on linguistics and syntax, and matched the trigger words in the dictionary with the help of syntactic dependency relations to get the trigger word types.

The rule-based approach is easy to understand. The disadvantage is that these methods rely on rules made by domain experts based on their expertise too much, which are only suitable for application in fields where knowledge is slowly updated. However, the knowledge in the field of biology updates rapidly, has many kinds, covers a wide range of information and spans a large span. Manual rule-making is difficult, which requires high expertise, consumes a lot of manpower, material resources and financial resources. It is difficult to rely on the rules to cover rich semantic information, and realize the trigger word detection of more literature materials. In addition, the generalization ability is poor and the recall rate is relatively low.

2.3 Machine Learning-Based Methods

The machine learning-based methods design features for labeled data, and employ machine learning models for multi-classification [11]. Common statistical machine learning models include: Support Vector Machine (SVM) [12], PA Online Algorithm [13], Bayesian Classifier, Markov Logic Network, Hidden Markov Logic Network [14], Maximum Entropy Markov Model, and Conditional Random Fields (CRF) [15], etc. SVM and CRF are widely used in biomedical trigger word detection.

The basic idea of SVM is to find a hyperplane with maximum interval for linearly separable tasks. Shen [4] used SVM to improve the objective function and increased the model attention to the corresponding features of a small number of samples, which not only balanced the accuracy rate and recall rate, but also improved the adaptability to multi-level and unbalanced corpus. The F1 value was 80.64% on the MLEE data set. Therefore, the sensitivities controllable support vector machine could alleviate the influence of unbalanced distribution of training samples labeled by different categories of biomedical events on trigger word recognition to a certain extent. He et al. [16] proposed a two-stage method based on SVM, which divided trigger detection into two stages: recognition and classification. They designed different features for each stage. The F1 value was 79.75% on the MLEE data set and 71.92% on the BioNLP09 data set respectively.

Huang et al. [17] used SVM method to predict drug interaction extraction based on features provided by recurrent neural network. Zhou et al. [18] used multi-kernel learning method, they employed one-to-many SVM to combine features embedded in neural language modeling with syntactic and semantic context features, then trained and tested the combined feature to classify trigger word. Sampo et al. [19] proposed a pipeline event extraction system EventMine based on SVM. The system consisted of four modules, each of which used one-to-one SVM to deal with the respective task as a multi-label classification problem. Zhou et al. [20] determined the distance between the sentences in the annotated corpus and the unannotated sentences by using the sentence structure and hidden topic, assigned event annotation to the unannotated sentences according to the distance automatically. They used sentences and newly assigned event annotations as well as annotated corpora to classify trigger words by one-to-many SVM. The idea of SVM classification is simple and the classification effect is good. However, the SVM algorithm is difficult to implement for large-scale training samples, it can not solve the problem of multi-classification, lack of data sensitivity.

CRF can model the target sequence based on the observed sequence, and focus on solving the problem of sequence annotation. Wang et al. [21] used Long Short Term memory (LSTM) network and CRF to detect trigger words, evaluated the influence of different word vectors on their models. They regarded the trigger words recognition as a sequence labeling problem, and improved the recognition accuracy of multi-word trigger words. According to different influence of features on different types of event trigger words, Wei et al. [22] proposed a hybrid CRF model which was based on CRF model and combined with the Brown Cluster method. Zhou et al. [23] regarded trigger word recognition as a sequence labeling problem, introduced BIO tag, and used maximum entropy Markov model to detect trigger words. The advantage of CRF model is that it can use the relationship between context markers to calculate the global parameter optimization, and the disadvantage is that the convergence speed is slow.

Compared with the methods based on dictionary and rules, the machine learning-based approaches save manual cost, which have better overall comprehensive effect and high popularization. In addition, they have low requirements on the integrity of semantic information and fast response speed. However, the traditional machine learning methods need to manually construct a large number of complex features. On the one hand, they are time consuming and costly. On the other hand, when the NLP tool is used to construct features manually, the cascaded errors of the NLP tool may lead to incorrect feature extraction and poor standardization. In a word, it is difficult to rely on manual to obtain large-scale, high-quality labeled data and effective features, and the generalization ability of the model is insufficient.

2.4 Deep Learning-Based Methods

The essence of deep learning method is a multi-layer representation learning method, which is an algorithm for abstract representation of data by using neural network structure including multi-layer nonlinear transformation. Deep learning-based methods have been widely applied in various fields, which have greatly promoted the development of artificial intelligence. In recent years, various deep learning methods based on word vectors and neural networks have been proposed successively. Common neural network models include: Convolutional Neural Network (CNN) [24], Recurrent Neural Network (RNN) [25], Long Short Term Memory Network (LSTM) [26], and Gated Recurrent Unit (GRU) [27], etc.

CNN is a kind of feedforward neural network with deep structure and convolution computation, which can carry out supervised learning and unsupervised learning. Qin [28] proposed a trigger word detection model based on parallel multi-pooling convolution neural network. It selected word vectors based on dependency relations, automatically extracted rich deep features such as sentence combination semantics through parallel convolution operations and processed multi-event sentences by dynamic multi-pooling operations. The F1 value of this method was 80.27% on the MLEE data set. It showed that the parallel operation of convolution pooling process with different window sizes could obtain rich semantic information between words, avoid relying on a large number of complex features design by hand, and improve the effect of trigger word recognition. Wang [29] proposed a biomedical event trigger word recognition model based on dynamic segmentation pooling CNN. The model performed convolution operations based on candidate trigger words and their features combined with contextual semantic information. The convolution result was subjected to a max-pooling according to the location of trigger words, and the sentence-level feature representation combined with the position information was obtained. The F1 value of this method was 78.31% on the MLEE data set. It showed that the dynamic segmented pooling CNN can effectively identify the types of trigger words by using location information, sentence structure and context features. Wang et al. [30] proposed a biomedical event trigger word detection method based on convolution neural network. Through the extensive embedding of semantic and syntactic information of words, the original input was transformed into a matrix. Then the matrix was input into CNN with multiple parallel convolution layers, combined with multiple low-level features to automatically extract global deep features for trigger word detection. Finally, the learned high-level feature representation was sent to the classifier based on neural network. Wang et al. [31] used different filters to obtain feature maps for getting deep features, and used CNN to unify the length of different distances between trigger words and candidate arguments. According to the dependence path between trigger words and candidate arguments, the sentence model was built, so as to detect the relationship between trigger word-argument or trigger word-trigger word. The pooling layer of CNN helped to reduce the parameters and computation in the network.

The advantage of CNN model is that it has fewer parameters and can learn and classify features simultaneously and optimize them globally. CNN has high robustness and fault tolerance. To some extent, CNN can alleviate the over-fitting problem caused by the unbalanced or small-scale training samples, improve the generalization ability of the model and the ability to adapt to the unbalanced samples. In addition, it can reduce the complexity of the model greatly. The disadvantage is that in CNN, information is transmitted in one direction, which mainly models the information in the local window. Convolution and pooling operation are used to extract local features, which cannot combine the overall sentence information such as context semantics and reference relation well, and it is difficult to model long-distance features.

RNN is a kind of recurrent neural network, which mainly learns the characteristics of samples and carries out supervised deep learning. Most RNN models are composed of directed connected units with memory and gating mechanisms, which input their current information and history information. Mikolov et al. [32] applied RNN in the field of natural language processing in 2010, and RNN had significant advantages in trigger word detection. Rahul [25] proposed a model based on Bi-directional cyclic neural network to extract high-level features at the sentence level. The model used RNN hidden layer state representation and word features to avoid complex artificial features generated by various NLP toolkits. Li et al. [33] regarded trigger word detection as a sequence labeling task, learned the features in the text through a bidirectional recurrent neural network, and generated the labels corresponding to the trigger words by CRF.

Compared with CNN modeling local information, RNN models sequence of indefinite length and better learns feature associations over long distances. RNN can utilize the timing information of sequential data, which is better than traditional feedforward neural networks. When the sequence length increases, the model based on RNN has obvious advantages over CNN. RNN has achieved great success in extracting temporal features and memory dependencies. However, when the learning sequence is too long, the information of the sequence text with a long distance from the current time accounts for less, the extraction ability is weak, and the serious gradient is easy to disappear. These may lead to the loss of long-distance information. At the same time, RNN depends on the activation function and grid parameters, which may cause gradient explosion and affect the accuracy seriously.

In order to avoid the influence of low accuracy caused by gradient disappearance and gradient explosion of RNN, LSTM is presented, which is a variant network structure of RNN. LSTM selectively weakens semantic information by forgetting information and enhances semantic information by retaining information [34], reduces information loss, effectively processes longer sequence input, and enhances the internal correlation of learning semantics. Jagannatha et al. [35] applied bidirectional LSTM to medical event detection in clinical medical records. Meng [1] constructed LKSIMP-BILSTM and LKSIMP-tree LSTM models respectively for temporal features of sentences and the dependency syntactic tree structure respectively. The F1 value of LKSFMP-BILSTM was 73.28% on the BioNLP11 data set and 72.22% on the BioNLP09 data set. LSTM can learn features automatically and has better data representation ability. He et al. [36] proposed a biomedical event trigger detection method based on BiLSTM, integrating attention mechanism and sentence embeddings. He [37] proposed a bidirectional LSTM triggered word recognition model based on sentence vector and word level attention mechanism. The model employed Bi-directional LSTM to enhance context feature representation, which could correlate more forward and backward information and ensure the integrity of information. Zhu et al. [38] converted trigger word recognition into sequence labeling task, used bidirectional LSTM to encode sentences into lists of hidden vectors, and assigned corresponding event labels to each word.

GRU is the variant of LSTM. GRU has two gating mechanisms, which combines the forgetting gate and the input gate of LSTM into a single update gate. Compared with LSTM, GRU has simpler structure, fewer model parameters, less over-fitting problem, faster convergence and faster training speed. Zhang [8] proposed a biomedical trigger word recognition model based on Bi-directional GRU model and self-attention mechanism. The model used the Bi-directional GRU model to obtain the sentence-level information such as the close context representation of the candidate trigger words, and captured the context sequence information to fully represent the sentence structure. The F1 value of this method was 80.31% on the MLEE data set. Li et al. [39] proposed a context tag sensitive gating network for biomedical event trigger words extraction. It captured context tag clues automatically, and introduced an GRU encoder based on attention mechanism to encode sentences. Bi-GRU captured the semantic information of each word effectively. The attention mechanism obtained more focused representation of information.

Compared with previous dictionary-based, rule-based and machine learning-based methods, deep learning methods utilize more semantic information, reduce the burden of manual feature design, and achieve better overall performance. Various neural network models learn the deep abstract continuous feature representation based on the original feature input automatically, which are more relevant to trigger word detection. They do not need to rely on manual construction of features, save time and effort, reduce the high requirement of domain specialization, and have high generalization. By adjusting the network parameters to automatically optimize and obtain the semantic features of the text, the ability of classification and prediction is improved, and the performance of identifying trigger words is improved. However, most of the trigger word detection models based on deep learning only use the information in the trigger word candidate and its surrounding local window, which lack complete and rich information to detect the trigger word. It is inevitable that the event type judgment error is caused by the polysemy of the trigger word. The neural network models have high requirements for the amount and distribution of training samples. If the data set size is too small or the data imbalance problem is too serious, the effect of deep learning will be affected.

2.5 Hybrid Models

In order to make full use of the advantages of various methods, hybrid models have been proposed to enhance their strengths and avoid weaknesses. Huang et al. [17] used LSTM and SVM to extract the relationship of drug side effects. They adopted a two-stage classification method. In the first stage, SVM was used for two classifications. In the second stage, LSTM was used to multi-classify the positive examples of the first stage. Shen [4] proposed a trigger word detection method based on attention mechanism and extreme learning machine. It only inputted a few general feature such as word representation, which did not construct features based on domain knowledge. The model mainly relied on CNN to alleviate the over-fitting problem caused by insufficient samples, and learnt the most relevant information about different types of triggers to obtain deep-seated features automatically by attention mechanism. It also used the extreme learning machine as the classifier to predict the trigger words according to the features. It had strong generalization ability and high prediction accuracy. The F1 value of this method was 81.5% on the BioNLP11 data set. Wang et al. [40] proposed a trigger word detection method based on Bi-directional LSTM and CRF. They regarded the trigger word detection as a sequence labeling problem, and used CRF to learn the global information effectively. The model did not design the initial complex feature engineering. It had strong ability of generalization. The bidirectional LSTM with large memory capacity was used to train character level embedding, which was combined with word level embedding to obtain a more effective word vector as the input of the next layer. The F1 value of this method was 78.08% on the MLEE data set.

The trigger word can be a single word or a phrasal verb with multiple words. The existing methods generally have poor performance in identifying multi-word trigger words. Wang [29] proposed a biological event trigger word recognition model based on BiLSTM-Attention-CRF hybrid model. The model transformed the task of trigger word recognition into a sequence tagging task, and used BIO tags to label samples, so as to make use of the correlation between sequence tags to improve the recognition ability of multi-word trigger words. The feature was constructed by BiLSTM, and the attention mechanism was added to assign the corresponding attention weight, which was convenient for CRF to label candidate trigger words. The F1 value of this method was 79.16% on the MLEE data set. It showed that the model was effective in detecting multi-word triggers. In addition, compared with the BiLSTM-CRF method without attention, the F1 value of this model increased by more than 0.5%, which indicated that the attention mechanism had a positive effect on the recognition of trigger words.

Depending on the context, the same word may have different meanings. In order to solve the problem of misjudgment of trigger word type and event type caused by polysemy, Wei [41] used three pre-trained language models (BioELMo, BioBERT and SCIBERT) as feature extractors to dynamically extract deep contextual word representations according to context. This model inputted rich semantic information of word vector into bidirectional LSTM for trigger word recognition and labels them with CRF. The F1 value of this method was 81.38% on the MLEE data set. Diao et al. [42] proposed a FBSN model to identify trigger word. FBSN was a hybrid structure composed of fine-grained bidirectional long short term memory network and SVM. FBi-LSTM was a BiLSTM network combining different levels of fine-grained representation, which could automatically extract deep high-level semantic features, reduce the difficulty and time cost of manual extraction of complex features. FBi-LSTM also used SVM to deal with small data sets and linear non-separable problems, so as to improve the classification performance. He et al. [43] proposed a hybrid neural network, which consisted of sliding window, multi-head attention, ReCNN and BiGRU. The problem of long-distance dependence could be handled by dividing long sentences into short sentences by using sliding windows. The model used ReCNN with strong learning local features to extract word-level features, integrated multi-head attention mechanism to enhance the key information and obtained the location information characteristics of each word. Their model introduces into BiGRU which obtains forward and backward information to train context information. The hybrid neural network of ReCNN and BiGRU solved the problem that traditional methods relied too much on tools for feature extraction. The F1 value of this method was 82.20% on the MLEE data set.

Zhu [11] regarded the trigger word recognition task as a multi-classification task, used natural language processing tools to extract the primary feature representation, and then employed BiLSTM to capture the context features so as to increase the sentence representation. GCN was used to model the syntactic structure obtained based on dependency parsing to further extract deeper structural features. Finally, Softmax function was used to complete the task of trigger word classification. This method did not need to design complex features manually. The F1 value of this method was 75.35% on the MLEE data set.

Tong [44] proposed a trigger word detection model based on Long Short Term Memory recurrent neural network and dynamic multi-pool convolution neural network. This model selected the basic features such as distributed semantic word vector features, and used LSTM to automatically extract and fully exploit the contextual information of text and the temporal features of sentences. This model did not need to design complex features manually, which used DMCNN to further learn the deep features so as to identify and classify the trigger words and event types.

Most of the neural network models for triggering word detection use sentence-level sequential modeling, which is inefficient in capturing long distance dependencies, and word vectors cannot fully capture the deep bidirectional features. In order to address these problems, Cheng et al. [45] proposed BGCN model. This model used BERT pre-trained model for large-scale training to capture contextual information and provide word vectors. This model introduced into syntactic analysis tree and used graph convolutional neural network to model syntactic, which further captured long-distance dependencies and enhanced the information representation of vectors. Finally, this model used a fully connected classification network to complete the recognition and classification prediction. On the ACE 2005 data set, the F1 value of the BGCN model was 77.6% on the trigger word recognition task and 74.2% on the trigger word classification task.

3   Data Set

The commonly used data set to detect trigger words include MLEE data set and BioNLP series data set, such as BioNLP09, BioNLP11, BioNLP13, and BioNLP16 data sets. MLEE data set is a general corpus in the field of biological information extraction, which contains molecular biological events represented by genes and proteins, as well as events of cellular, pathological, tissue and organ levels [11]. These events can be divided into 19 types, such as cell Proliferation, Regulation, Development, etc. Each event has a trigger word. MLEE data set contains independent training sets, development sets, and test sets. BioNLP data set contains 9 event types, including Gene Expression, Transcription and Protein Catabolism, which are designed to extract biological events on the molecular level. BioNLP data set mainly provides the training set and the development set, and adopts the way of online evaluation to predict and evaluate the test set [37]. MLEE data set and BioNLP data set are annotated in the same way. The static distribution of MLEE corpus and BioNLP11 are shown in Table 1 and Table 2.

Table 1. The static distribution of MLEE corpus

Data	Train	Devel	Test	Total
Document	131	44	87	262
Sentence	1271	457	880	2608
Event	3296	1175	2206	6677

Table 2. The static distribution of BioNLP11 corpus

Data	Train	Devel	Test
Document	800	150	260
Protein	9300	2080	3589
Event	8615	1795	3193
Word	176146	33827	57256

4   Current Problems and Future Development Trend

With the deepening of the research of natural language processing in the biomedical field, many scholars have proposed solutions to the problems faced in the task of biomedical event trigger word recognition. However, there is still a wide space for the development of trigger word recognition research. In view of the main problems, future research can be continued to explore from the following aspects.

(1) Improving the Generalization Ability
   Biomedical events have a wide range and span, however, the generalization ability of trigger word detection methods is generally insufficient. To address the problem, we can continue to explore domain feature independent event trigger word detection models that do not rely on artificially designed features, use deep learning neural networks to automatically learn features, employ machine learning models with strong predictive power as classifiers, and continue to explore trigger word detection methods that can be extended to many types of medical events methods.
(2) Alleviating the Imbalance of Data Sets.
   Data sparsity and data type imbalance are common problems in biomedical texts. In order to solve the problems, we can explore solutions from the aspects of sensitivity-controllable detection model, two-stage classification method and under sampling strategy in the future work. By using the method of two-stage classification, the influence of the imbalance of each classification data is less than that of one-stage classification. Using a machine learning model with controllable sensitivity as a classifier and changing the objective function can improve the effect of the trigger word recognition method in dealing with the unbalanced data set. According to the different categories of the sample corpus, the under sampling strategy can be used

to randomly remove some negative examples from the training samples and try a more targeted data balance adjustment method.

(3) Expanding the Scope of Research.

At present, the task of event extraction and trigger word recognition in biomedical field mainly focuses on biomedical literature. In the future, the research scope can be extended to biomedical events in texts on social media platforms such as Weibo, Baidu Q&A and electronic health records. In addition, more abundant domain knowledge can be obtained from other knowledge bases and knowledge maps to further improve the performance of trigger word recognition.

(4) Exploring New Methods

Aiming at the common problems of high manual labeling cost and few labeled samples in the biomedical field, we can learn the methods in different research fields, such as generating countermeasure network, remote supervision method, inverse reinforcement learning, small sample learning, dynamic reward mechanism and so on. Meanwhile, we also need to combine with the characteristics and needs of the biomedical field to study new methods that can generalize to different tasks in the biomedical field.

(5) Exploring Joint Extraction.

Biomedical events are mainly composed of trigger words and arguments. Most of the existing event extraction methods adopt pipeline mode: identify the trigger word first, then detect the arguments. It not only ignores the connection between trigger words and arguments, but also easily causes cascade errors. There are relatively few existing models based on joint event extraction. In the future work, we can try the joint extraction method based on deep learning to model the overall structure of biomedical events, extract and identify trigger words and arguments at the same time, and correct each other to achieve information complementarity and feature sharing. In addition, we can try to build a synonym thesaurus to enrich features.

(6) Improving the Extraction Performance of Complex Events.

As the composition of complex events is more complex, there are usually many elements, and there exist nested events, which makes the complex event is difficult to identify. Therefore, the extraction performance of complex events is much lower than that of simple events in event trigger word recognition. How to build a better model for complex events needs further exploration.

5 Conclusion

With the continuous advancement of biomedical research in recent years, biomedical literature has increased rapidly. Extracting data from biomedical literature has become an important research subject in the field of natural language processing. Biomedical event extraction is helpful to mining biomedical information conveniently. Trigger word detection is the basic segment of event extraction. The performance of trigger word detection has a great influence on the effect of event extraction. In this paper, we firstly introduce the background, concept, goal and significance of biomedical event trigger word detection, then summarize the existing methods of trigger word recognition, their advantages and disadvantages, and their application. Finally, we analyze the problems and challenges in the existing work, and look forward to the future research direction and development trend.

Acknowledgement. This work was supported by the National Natural Science Foundation of China (No. 62006108, No. 61976109), General program of China Postdoctoral Science Foundation (No. 2022M710593), Natural Science research projects of Liaoning Education Department (No. LQ2020027), Liaoning Provincial Science and Technology Fund project (No. 2021-BS-201), Innovative Talent Support Program of Liaoning Province, Liaoning Provincial Key Laboratory Special Fund, Dalian Key Laboratory Special Fund.

References

1. Meng, T.: Research on biomedical event extraction based on domain semantic information. Master's thesis of Tianjin University (2020)
2. Ananiadou, S., Thompson, P., Nawaz, R., McNaught, J., Kell D.B.: Event based text mining for biology and functional genomics. Brief. Funct. Genomics **14**(3), 213–230 (2015)
3. Sampo, P., Tomoko, O., Rafal, R., Andrew, R., Hong-Woo, C., Sung-Jae, J., et al.: Overview of the cancer genetics and pathway curation tasks of BioNLP shared task 2013. BMC Bioinform. **16**(S10), S2 (2015)
4. Shen, C.: Research on detecting biomedical event and its trigger. Doctoral thesis of Dalian University of Technology (2021)
5. Zhang, J., Liu, M., Zhang, Y.: Topic informed neural approach for biomedical event extraction. Artif. Intell. Med. **103**(C), 101783 (2020)
6. Buyko, E., Faessler, E., Wermter, J., Hahn, U.: Event extraction from trimmed dependency graphs. In: Bionlp Proceedings of the Workshop on Current Trends in Biomedical Natural Language Processing, pp. 19–27 (2009)
7. Bronstein, O., Dagan, I., Li, Q., Ji, H., Frank, A.: Seed-based event trigger labeling: how far can event descriptions get us? In: Proceedings of the 53rd Annual Meeting of the Association for Computational Linguistics and the 7th International Joint Conference on Natural Language Processing, no. 2, pp. 372–376 (2015)
8. Zhang, R.: Research on biomedical event extraction technology. Master's thesis of Northwest Normal University (2020)
9. Minh, Q.L., Truong, S.N, Bao, Q.H.: A pattern approach for biomedical event annotation. In: Bionlp Shared Task 2011 Workshop, Portland, Oregon, USA, pp. 149–150 (2011)
10. Kilicoglu, H., Bergler, S.: Adapting a general semantic interpretation approach to biological event extraction. In: Bionlp Shared Task 2011 Workshop, Portland, Oregon, pp. 173–182 (2011)
11. Zhu, L.: Research and implementation of biomedical event extraction method. Master's thesis of Nanjing Normal University (2020)
12. Cortes, C., Vapnik, V.: Support vector networks. Mach. Learn. **20**(3), 273–297 (1995)
13. Crammer, K., Dekel, O., Keshet, J., Shalev-Shwartz, S., Singer, Y.: Online passive-aggressive algorithms. J. Mach. Learn. Res. **7**(3), 551–585 (2006)
14. Baum, L.E., Petrie, T.: Statistical inference for probabilistic functions of finite state Markov chains. Ann. Math. Stat. **37**(6), 1554–1563 (1966)
15. Lafferty, J.D., Mccallum, A., Pereira, F.C.N.: Conditional random fields: probabilistic models for segmenting and labeling sequence data. In: Proceedings of the Eighteenth International Conference on Machine Learning, Williamstown, MA, USA, pp. 282–289 (2001)

16. He, X., Li, L., Liu, Y., Yu, X., Meng, J.: A two-stage biomedical event trigger detection method integrating feature selection and word embeddings. IEEE/ACM Trans. Comput. Biol. Bioinform. **15**(4), 1325–1332 (2018)
17. Huang, D., Jiang, Z., Zou, L., Li, L.: Drug-drug interaction extraction from biomedical literature using suppport vector machine and long short term memory networks. Inf. Sci. **415**, 100–109 (2017)
18. Zhou, D., Zhong, D., He, Y.: Event trigger identification for biomedical events extraction using domain knowledge. Bioinformatics **30**(11), 1587–1594 (2014)
19. Sampo, P., Tomoko, O., Makoto, M., Han-Cheol, C., Jun'ichi, T., Sophia, A.: Event extraction across multiple levels of biological organization. Bioinformatics **28**(18), 575–581 (2012)
20. Zhou, D., Zhong, D.: A semi-supervised learning framework for biomedical event extraction based on hidden topics. Artif. Intell. Med. **64**(1), 51–58 (2015)
21. Wang, Y., Wang, J., Lin, H., Zhang, S., Li, L.: Bomedical event trigger detection based on bidrectional LSTM and CRF. In: 2017 IEEE International Conference on Bioinformatics and Biomedicine (BIBM), pp. 445–450. IEEE (2017)
22. Wei, X., Huang, Y., Chen, B., Ji, D.: Research on tagging biomedical event trigger. Comput. Sci. **42**(10), 239–243 (2015)
23. Zhou, D., He, Y.: Biomedical events extraction using the hidden vector state model. Artif. Intell. Med. **53**(3), 205–213 (2011)
24. Collobert, R., Weston, J., Bottou, L., Karlen, M., Kavukcuoglu, K., Kuksa, P.: Natural language processing from scratch. J. Mach. Learn. Res. **12**(1), 2493–2537 (2011)
25. Rahul, P.V.S.S., Sahu, S.K., Anand, A.: Biomedical event trigger identification using bidirectional recurrent neural network based models. arXiv preprint arXiv.1705.09516 (2017)
26. Hochreiter, S., Schmidhuber, J.: Long short-term memory. Neural Comput. **9**, 1735–1780 (1997)
27. Cho, K., Merrienboer, B.V., Gulcehre, C., Bahdanau, D., Bougares, F., Schwenk, H., et al.: Learning phrase representations using RNN encoder-decoder for statistical machine translation. In: Proceedings of the 2014 Conference on Empirical Methods in Natural Language Processing (EMNLP), Doha, Qatar, pp. 1724–1734 (2014)
28. Qin, M.: Extracting biomedical events with parallel multi-pooling convolutional neural network. Master's thesis of Dalian University of Technology (2017)
29. Wang, A.: Biomedical information extraction based on event framework. Master's thesis of Dalian University of Technology (2018)
30. Wang, J., Li, H., An, Y., Lin, H., Yang, Z.: Biomedical event trigger detection based on convolutional neural network. Int. J. Data Min. Bioinform. **15**(3), 195–213 (2016)
31. Wang, A., Jian, W., Lin, H., Zhang, J., Yang, Z., Xu, K.: A multiple distributed representation method based on neural network for biomedical event extraction. BMC Med. Inform. Decis. Mak. **17**(3), 171–179 (2017)
32. Mikolov, T., Karafiát, M., Burget, L., Cernocký, J., Khudanpur, S.: Recurrent neural network based language model. In: 11th Annual Conference of the International Speech Communication Association, Makuhair, Chiba, Japan, pp. 1045–1048 (2010)
33. Li, L., Liu, Y.: Exploiting argument information to improve biomedical event trigger identification via recurrent neural networks and supervised attention mechanisms. In: 2017 IEEE International Conference on Bioinformatics and Biomedicine (BIBM), pp. 565–568 (2017)
34. Yan, S., Wong, K.-C.: Context awareness and embedding for biomedical event extraction. Bioinformatics **36**(2), 637–643 (2020)
35. Jagannatha, A.N., Yu, H.: Bidirectional RNN for medical event detection in electronic health records. In: Proceedings of the 2016 Conference of the North American Chapter of the Association for Computational Linguistics: Human Language Technologies, pp. 473–482 (2016)

36. He, X., Li, L., Wan, J., Song, D., Meng, J., Wang Z.: Biomedical event trigger detection based on BiLSTM integrating attention mechanism and sentence vector. In: 2018 IEEE International Conference on Bioinformatics and Biomedicine (BIBM), pp. 651–654 (2018)
37. He, X.: Research on the main issues of biological event extraction based on text mining. Doctoral thesis of Dalian University of Technology (2019)
38. Zhu, L., Zheng, H.: Biomedical event extraction with a novel combination strategy based on hybrid deep neural networks. BMC Bioinform. **21**(1), 47 (2020)
39. Li, L., Huang, M., Liu, Y., Qian, S., He, X.: Contextual label sensitive gated network for biomedical event trigger extraction. J. Biomed. Inform. **95**, 103221 (2019)
40. Wang, Y., Wang, J., Lin, H., Tang, X., Zhang, S., Li, L.: Bidirectional long short-term memory with CRF for detecting biomedical event trigger in fast text semantic space. BMC Bioinform. **19**(Suppl. 20), 507 (2018)
41. Wei, Y.: Research on biomedical event extraction method based on pre-training language model. Master's Thesis of Wuhan University of Science and Technology. (2020)
42. Diao, Y., Lin, H., Yang, L., Fan, X., Wu, D., Yang, Z., et al.: FBSN: a hybrid fine-grained neural network for biomedical event trigger identification. Neurocomputing **381**(C), 105–112 (2019)
43. He, X., Yu, B., Ren, Y.: SWACG: a hybrid neural network integrating sliding window for biomedical event trigger extraction. J. Imaging Sci. Technol. **65**(6), 060502-1–060502-13 (2021)
44. Tong, J.: Biomedical event extraction mechanism based on combinatorial deep learning. Master's thesis of Wuhan University of Science and Technology (2018)
45. Cheng, S., Ge, W., Wang, Y., XU, J.: BGCN: trigger detection based on Bert and graph convolution network. Comput. Sci. **48**(7), 292–298 (2021)

BG-INT: An Entity Alignment Interaction Model Based on BERT and GCN

Yu Song[1], Mingyu Gui[1], Chenxin Hu[1,3], Kunli Zhang[1,2(✉)], Shuai Zhang[1], and Wenxuan Zhang[1]

[1] College of Computer and Artificial Intelligence, Zhengzhou University, Zhengzhou, China
{ieysong,ieklzhang}@zzu.edu.cn
[2] Pengcheng Laboratory, Shenzhen, Guangdong, China
[3] He'nan Cancer Hospital/Affiliated Cancer Hospital of Zhengzhou University, Zhengzhou, China

Abstract. Knowledge fusion can complementarily integrate knowledge in multi-source knowledge graphs, and is a key step in building knowledge graphs, where multi-source data includes monolingual and multilingual data. Entity alignment is a key technology for knowledge fusion, while existing entity alignment models only use entity part information to learn vector representations, which limits the performance of the models. This paper proposes an entity alignment interaction model based on BERT and GCN - BG-INT. The model learns entity embeddings from entity names/descriptions, relationships, attributes, and graph structures, and makes full use of all aspects of entity information for entity alignment. Experiments on the public multilingual dataset DBP15K show that BG-INT outperforms existing models in entity alignment. In addition, on the multi-source monolingual cardiovascular and cerebrovascular dataset, the HitRatio@1 of BG-INT also reaches 96.5%, and 2840 pieces of cardiovascular and cerebrovascular data redundancy are eliminated after knowledge fusion. We propose an entity interaction model based on BERT and GCN, and demonstrate the effectiveness of the proposed model on the multilingual dataset DBP15K and the monolingual cardiovascular and cerebrovascular dataset.

Keywords: Knowledge fusion · Entity alignment · BERT · Graph convolutional network · Knowledge graph construction

1 Introduction

Knowledge fusion refers to the process of fusing information such as different concepts, contexts, and different expressions from multiple sources. Knowledge fusion technology can provide an effective extension method for the constructed knowledge graph (KG) or knowledge resources to complete knowledge update or supplement, thus improving the knowledge coverage. It can also eliminate the ambiguities and inconsistencies among entities, concepts, and semantic relationships in multiple sources, thus creating prerequisites for the construction of knowledge graph.

B. Tang et al. (Eds.): CHIP 2022, CCIS 1772, pp. 67–81, 2023.
https://doi.org/10.1007/978-981-19-9865-2_5

In the process of knowledge fusion, the main work involved is Entity Alignment (EA). EA is the process of judging whether two entities in different sources point to the same object in the real world. If multiple entities represent the same object, an alignment relationship is constructed between these entities, and the information contained in the entities is fused and aggregated at the same time. In KG from different sources, aligned entities are connected by Inter-Lingual Links (ILLs), as shown at the top of Fig. 1. However, the coverage of ILLs in existing KGs is rather low [4]: for example, less than 20% of entities in DBpedia are covered by ILLs. The goal of EA is to find the missing ILLs in the KG.

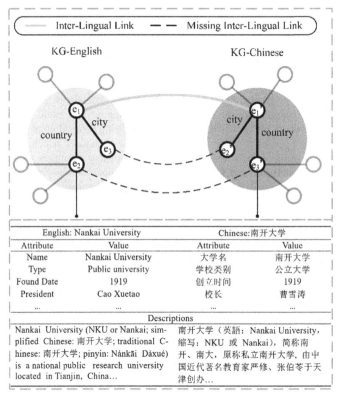

Fig. 1. Example snippet of two KGs (English and Chinese) connected by interlingual links (ILLs) in the DBP15K [1] dataset.

In the past few years, many EA techniques employ deep learning methods to learn efficient vector representations (i.e., embedding representations), and then perform EA based on the vector representations. Specific techniques include translation-based embedding models, such as MTransE proposed by Chen et al. [3] to unify different KGs into the same low-dimensional vector space, which only uses KG graph structure information as the feature of vector representation. MultiKE proposed by Zhang et al. [4] and AttrE proposed by Trisedya et al. [5] exploit the graph structure information and also combine a total of four types of raw information, relational predicates, attribute predicates, and attribute values, as input features for the training and alignment modules to obtain better performance. In recent years, embedding models based on graph neural network(GNN) have also been used for EA. While the variant of graph neural network, the graph convolutional network (GCN) [6], has achieved state-of-the-art results in various graph applications, such as GCN-Align [7], HMAN [8], HGCN [9], RDGCN [10], SSP [11], NMN [12], CEA [13], DINGAL[14] and other GCN-based models have been proposed to achieve good results in EA tasks. Among them, the HMAN model proposed by Yang et al. [8] uses attribute values and entity descriptions as input features to correct the learned vector representation based on capturing the structural features of the graph, and obtains better performance.

In addition to side information such as graph structure, relationships, and attributes, entities also contain rich literal descriptions [2], as shown at the bottom of Fig. 1. The above models only use part of the information of the entity to learn the vector representation. For example, AttrE [5] does not use the description information of the entity, and HMAN does not use the relationship information of the entity, which limits the performance of EA to a certain extent. Therefore, to take full advantage of all aspects of entity information to learn effective vector representations, this paper combines the use of graph convolutional networks (GCNs) to capture entity graphs based on the BERT-INT [17] model that utilizes side information for EA. Structural information, a BERT and GCN-based EA interaction model - BG-INT is proposed. The main contributions of this paper are as follows:

1) An EA model BG-INT (EA Interaction Model Based on BERT and GCN, BG-INT) is proposed, which fully utilizes all aspects of entity information (graph structure, name/description, relationship, attribute) to learn effective vector representation. On the multilingual dataset DBP15K, the BG-INT model outperforms the state-of-the-art model by 0.1%–0.6% in HitRatio@1.
2) The BG-INT model is used to fuse the cardiovascular and cerebrovascular disease datasets from multiple sources, of which HitRatio@1 reached 96.5%, eliminating 2840 pieces of cardiovascular and cerebrovascular data redundancy.

2 Problem Definition

Definition 1: KG. Define KG as $G = \{E, R, A, V, D\}$ and KG' as $G' = \{E', R', A', V', D'\}$. Take KG as an example, where E, R, A, V, D represents a collection of entities, relationships, attributes, attribute values, and entity descriptions, respectively. For each $e \in E, r \in R, a \in A, v \in V, d \in D$ represents an entity, relationship, attribute, attribute value and entity description. For KG contains relation triples (h, r, t) and attribute triples (h, a, v), where $h, r \in E, r \in R, a \in A, v \in V$. In addition, KG also contains entity description dyads (h, d_h) and (t, d_t), where $d_h, d_t \in D$.

Definition 2: EA. Given two KGs KG and KG' and a set of prealigned entity pair seeds $I = \{(e \sim e')\}$, the goal is to learn a ranking function $f: E \times E' \to \mathbb{R}$ to compute the similarity score between two entities, based on which the correctly aligned entities e' With any queried entity e is ranked as high as possible among all entities in E'.

3   BG-INT Model

The BG-INT model is shown in Fig. 2, which includes two parts: an embedding unit
and an interaction unit. The embedding unit is the basis of the interaction unit, which
is composed of BERT and GCN. BERT is mainly used as the name, description, and
neighbor entity of the embedded entity, and GCN is mainly the basic representation
unit of the graph structure. The interaction unit is used to compute the interactions
between the embeddings learned from the embedding unit, including name/description-
view interaction, neighbor-view interaction, and attribute-view interaction.

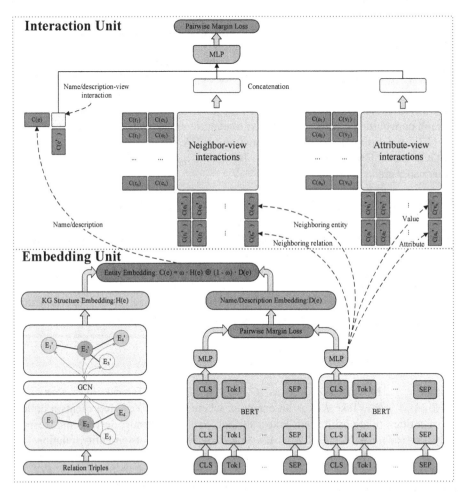

Fig. 2. The overall framework of the BG-INT model.

3.1 Embedding Unit

This unit learns entity name/description, relation, and attribute embeddings by fine-tuning the pre-trained model BERT, applies GCNs to learn entity graph structure embeddings, and forms preliminary entity embeddings after weighted concatenation of entity name/description and graph structure embeddings.

BERT. The pre-training model BERT (Bidirectional Encoder Representation from Transformers) can obtain word meanings based on the context of the sentence, while being able to extract relational features at several different levels, thus reflecting the sentence semantics more comprehensively. In addition, the text descriptions of the two equivalent entities are semantically similar. Therefore, when learning entity embedding from the aspect of name/description, the entity description should be used preferentially, because the entity description contains more rich information than the entity name, and the name is used instead when the entity lacks the corresponding description.

Specifically, we use two BERT basic units to compose the PAIRWISEBERT model. The model uses the entity name/description as its input, the input is of the form [CLS] $e(e')$ [SEP] or [CLS] $d(d')$ [SEP], let the input be encoded in PAIRWISEBERT, select the hidden state of [CLS] as the entity name/ The text embedding of the description is used for training. After filtering the CLS embedding of PAIRWISEBERT through the MLP layer, the entity name/description embedding is obtained:

$$D(e) = MLP(CLS(e)) \tag{1}$$

In addition, we use random uniform negative sampling to construct the training dataset $T = \{(e, e'^+, e'^-)\}$ to optimize the loss function afterward, which represents the entity being queried, and $e'^+, e'^- \in E'$ represents the positive samples aligned with e and the unaligned negative samples, respectively. To embed the text of entity names/descriptions into the same vector space, we fine-tune the PAIRWISEBERT model with a pairwise marginal loss L:

$$L = \sum_{(e,e'^+,e'^-)\in T} \max\{0, g(e, e'^+) - g(e, e'^-) + m\} \tag{2}$$

where m is the distance boundary value between positive samples and negative samples, and $g(e, e')$ is the instantiated ℓ_1 distance used to measure the similarity between $D(e)$ and $D(e')$.

GCN. Graph convolutional network GCNs (Graph Convolutional Networks) is a neural network that directly operates on graph data, and its essence is to extract the structural features of graphs. Since the structural information of equivalent entities in KGs is also similar, GCNs can exploit the structural information of KGs to learn entity embeddings. Meanwhile, Wang et al. used GCNs to embed entities into a unified vector space and achieved remarkable performance in EA. We therefore utilize GCNs to map entities into a low-dimensional vector space where equivalent entities are close to each other to obtain embeddings in terms of the entity graph structure.

The GCN model consists of multiple stacked GCN layers. The input of the l layer of the GCN model is a vertex feature matrix $\mathbf{H}^{(l)} \in \mathbb{R}^{n*d(l)}$, where n is the number of vertices and $d^{(l)}$ is the number of features in the l layer. The output of layer l is a new feature matrix $\mathbf{H}^{(l+1)}$, which is calculated by convolution with the following formula:

$$\mathbf{H}^{(l+1)} = \sigma(\tilde{\boldsymbol{D}}^{-\frac{1}{2}} \tilde{\mathbf{A}} \tilde{\mathbf{D}}^{-\frac{1}{2}} \mathbf{H}^{(l)} \mathbf{W}^{(l)}) \tag{3}$$

Among them, l is the number of GCN layers, $\mathbf{H}$ is the feature of each layer, $\sigma(\cdot)$ is the nonlinear activation function, $\mathbf{A}$ is the $n * n$ dimensional connectivity matrix, also known as the adjacency matrix, which represents the structural information of the graph, $\tilde{A} = \mathbf{A} + \mathbf{I}$, $\mathbf{I}$ is the identity matrix, $\tilde{\boldsymbol{D}}$ is the degree matrix of $\tilde{A}$, $\mathbf{W}^{(l)} \in \mathbb{R}^{d^{(l)}*d^{(l+1)}}$ represents the weight matrix of the l layer in GCN, and $d^{(l+1)}$ is the dimension of the new vertex feature.

In the BG-INT model, we use GCNs to embed entities in different KGs into a unified vector space based on the information on the graph structure of KGs. Specifically, the BG-INT model uses two two-layer GCNs, named GCN1 and GCN2, to learn structural embeddings that propagate neighbor entity information in the two KGs, respectively. For the structural feature vector of the entity, the dimension of the structural feature vector is defined as d_s in each GCN, the weight matrices of the two layers in the two GCNs are defined as $\mathbf{W}_s^{(1)}$ and $\mathbf{W}_s^{(2)}$ respectively, and GCN1 and GCN2 share $\mathbf{W}_s^{(1)}$ and $\mathbf{W}_s^{(2)}$, The structural feature matrices of each GCN input are defined as $\mathbf{H}_s^{(0)}$ and $\mathbf{H}_{s'}^{(0)}$, respectively, the structural embeddings at the output are defined as $\mathbf{H}_s^{(2)}$ and $\mathbf{H}_{s'}^{(2)}$. The final learned entity graph structure embedding is denoted as $H(e)$.

Weighted Connection. The name/description embedding learned by BERT is denoted as $D(e)$, and the graph structure embedding learned by GCN is denoted as $H(e)$. A simple way to combine these two modules is through weighted connection, as shown in Equation:

$$C(e) = \tau \cdot D(e) \oplus (1 - \tau) \cdot H(e) \tag{4}$$

where τ is a weight hyperparameter that balances name/description embeddings and text embeddings. $C(e)$ represents the final entity embedding after weighted connection.

3.2 Interaction Unit

Based on the embedding unit, an interaction model consisting of name/description view interaction, neighbor view interaction and attribute view interaction is established.

Name/Description View Interaction. We get the final e and e' name/description embeddings $C(e)$ and $C(e')$ from the embedding unit, and then compute their cosine similarity $\cos(C(e), C(e'))$ as the result of the name/description view interaction.

Neighbor View Interaction. We establish the interaction between neighbors $N(e)$ and $N(e')$. The general idea is to compare the name/description of each neighbor pair instead of learning a global representation of e or e' by aggregating the names/descriptions of all neighbors.

Specifically, firstly, given two entities e and e' in KG and KG', calculate the name/description vector representation of e and e' neighbors and the relationship vector representation between neighbors according to formula (1), and obtain four sets of directions $\{C(e_i)\}_{i=1}^{|N(e)|}$, $\{C(e'_j)\}_{j=1}^{|N(e)|}$, $\{C(r_i)\}_{i=1}^{|N(e)|}$, and $\{C(r'_j)\}_{j=1}^{|N(e)|}$, then use the cosine similarity to calculate the similarity matrix $\mathbf{S}$ of the neighbor's name/description vector set, where the elements are $s_{ij} = sim(C(e_i), C(e'_j))$, and use the relationship with the neighbors to calculate the mask matrix $\mathbf{M}$, where the elements are $m_{ij} = sim(C(r_i), C(r'_j))$, Then use $\mathbf{M}$ to correct $\mathbf{S}$, that is, $S_{ij} = S_{ij} \otimes M_{ij}$, where $\otimes$ is the multiplication operation between elements, finally, use the double aggregation function to calculate the corrected $\mathbf{S}$, and obtain the neighbor view interaction vector, which is the result of neighbor view interaction.

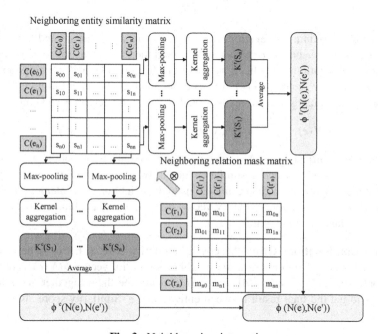

Fig. 3. Neighbor view interaction.

The double aggregation function is to aggregate from the row direction and column direction of the matrix $\mathbf{S}$ respectively, and finally splice the aggregation result vectors in the two directions. Taking row aggregation as an example, first perform the maximum pooling operation on the similarity matrix $\mathbf{S}$, as shown in formula (5):

$$s_i^{max} = \max_{j=0}^{n}\{s_{i0}, \cdots, s_{ij}, \cdots, s_{in}\}. \tag{5}$$

Then use the Gaussian kernel function to perform a one-to-many mapping on s_i^{max} to obtain multiple mapping values to form a vector $\mathbf{K}^r(\mathbf{S}_i)$, as shown in formula (6):

$$K_l(s_i^{max}) = \exp\left[-\frac{(s_i^{max}-\mu_l)^2}{2\sigma_l^2}\right],$$
$$\mathbf{K}^r(\mathbf{S}_i) = [K_1(s_i^{max}), \cdots, K_l(s_i^{max}), \cdots, K_L(s_i^{max})]. \tag{6}$$

Finally, all $\mathbf{K}^r(\mathbf{S}_i)$ are paired in the row direction Average of numbers to get a row aggregate vector $\phi^r(N(e), N(e'))$ of length L. The formula to achieve row aggregation is shown in formula (7):

$$\phi^r(N(e), N(e')) = \frac{1}{|N(e)|}\sum_{i=1}^{|N(e)|} \log \mathbf{K}^r(\mathbf{S}_i). \tag{7}$$

The steps of column aggregation are similar to row aggregation, and the obtained column aggregation vector is $\phi^c(N(e), N(e'))$, and then the results of row aggregation and column aggregation are spliced according to formula (4), and the neighbor view interaction similarity vector $\phi(N(e), N(e'))$ is obtained, as shown in formula (8), where $\oplus$ represents the splicing operation, and Fig. 3 below is the neighbor view interaction.

$$\phi(N(e), N(e')) = \phi^r(N(e), N(e')) \oplus \phi^c(N(e), N(e')) \tag{8}$$

Attribute View Interaction. An attribute triple of entities e and e' is (e, a_i, v_i), (e', a_j', v_j'), respectively, which is similar to the entity's neighbor relationship triple, so the attribute view interaction can be analogous to the neighbor view interaction. Finally, the attribute-view interaction similarity vector $\phi(A(e), A(e'))$ is obtained, which is the result of attribute-view interaction.

The Final Combination. Given the cosine similarity $\cos(C(e), C(e'))$ between the descriptions/names of two entities, the neighbor similarity vector $\phi(N(e), N(e'))$ and the attribute similarity vector $\phi(A(e), A(e'))$, concatenate them together and apply an MLP layer to get the final result between entity e and e' Similarity score, as shown in formula:

$$\phi(e, e') = [\phi(N(e), N(e')) \oplus \phi(A(e), A(e'))$$
$$\oplus \cos(C(e), C(e'))], \tag{9}$$
$$g(e, e') = \text{MLP}(\phi(e, e')).$$

3.3 Entity Alignment

The embedding of each entity is first obtained by Eq. (4) using the BERT. Then calculate the cosine similarity between e of the embeddings in KG and all e' of the embeddings in KG', and return $top-\kappa$ similar entities as e candidates according to the cosine similarity. Finally, for e and each candidate, an interaction model is used to calculate the similarity score between them, and all candidates are ranked from large to small for evaluation according to the similarity score.

4   Experiments

This section introduces the EA experiments of the BG-INT model in the DBP15K and cardiovascular and cerebrovascular dataset (CCDataset), and validates the effectiveness of the BG-INT model through the experimental results. The metrics are HitRatio@K (K = 1, 10) and MRR (refer to Sun et al. [15] for details).

4.1   Data Preparation

This section introduces the construction process of CCDataset. As shown in Fig. 4, the process can be divided into the formulation of cardiovascular and cerebrovascular labeling specifications, and the labeling and processing of corpus. For the formulation of labeling specifications, first collect international standard medical terminology and case labeling and analysis to design a concept classification system and a relationship classification system, and then further improve the system specification after evaluation by medical experts to form a corpus labeling system and use it to guide manual and Automatic labeling. The labeling and processing process of corpus first collects multi-source cardiovascular and cerebrovascular medical data, extracts unstructured or semi-structured text data, and then starts manual and automatic labeling after corpus preprocessing, and then corpus post-processing stage, and finally form a CCDataset.

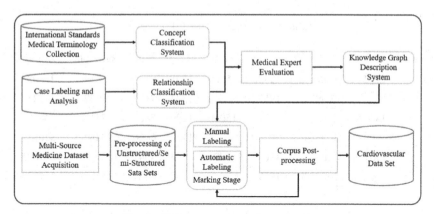

Fig. 4. CCDataset construction process.

The sources of knowledge related to cardiovascular and cerebrovascular diseases are different. As shown in Table 1, unstructured data comes from websites or medical guide software, such as clinical guide APPs[1] and medical search website[2]. Semi-structured data comes from medical textbooks, clinical Medical guidelines, etc., the structured data comes from CMeKG[3] (Chinese Medical KG), CSKB (Chinese Medical Symptom Knowledge Base) and CMKB[16] (Chinese Medical Drug Knowledge Base).

---

[1] http://guide.medlive.cn/.

[2] https://www.xywy.com/.

[3] http://cmekg.pcl.ac.cn/.

Table 1. Statistical results of cardiovascular and cerebrovascular data sources.

Source	Type	Size
Medical textbooks	Semi-structured/Unstructured	6,001,580 words
Medical guidelines	Semi-structured/Unstructured	247,358 words
Seek medical advice	Unstructured	5,539 articles
CMeKG	Structured	6,493 articles
CSKB	Structured	1,725 articles
CMKB	Structured	12,736 articles

4.2 Dataset and Parameter Settings

Dataset. The dataset uses the multilingual DBP15K dataset and the monolingual CCDataset.

The data statistics of the DBP15K dataset used in this experiment are shown in Table 2 below. DBP15K contains three subsets of ZH-EN, JA-EN and FR-EN. Each subset contains 15,000 reference EAs. After dividing the training set and test set by 3:7, the training set is 4500 and the test set is 10500.

Table 2. Statistics of DBP15K dataset.

Datasets			Ent	ILLS	Rel.	Attr.	Rel.triples	Attr.triples
DBP15K	ZH-EN	Chinese	19388	15000	1701	8111	70414	248035
		English	19572		1323	7173	95142	343218
	JA-EN	Japanese	19814	15000	1299	5882	77214	248991
		English	19780		1153	6066	93484	320616
	FR-EN	French	19661	15000	903	4547	105998	273825
		English	19993		1208	6422	115722	351094

This experiment needs to perform knowledge fusion operation for cardiovascular and cerebrovascular data, so data in different texts should be labeled and machine extracted. Table 3 below is the data statistics of CCDataset. The KG G is the manually labeled dataset, and the KG G′ is the model labeled dataset. The weighted similarity of entities between KG G and KG G′ is pre-computed using Jaccrad, longest common subsequence, and Levenshtein to find linked entity pairs for later model training and testing. The total number of entity links finally obtained is 693. After dividing the training set and the test set according to 3:7, the training set is 210 and the test set is 483.

Table 3. Quantitative statistics of CCDataset.

G			G′		
Ent.	Rel.	Rel.triples	Ent.	Rel.	Rel.triples
9561	99	15258	15199	42	34051

Parameter Settings. In the embedding unit, the CLS embedding dimension of the BERT is 768, and we use a 300-dimensional MLP in formula (1) to obtain a lower-dimensional CLS embedding. At the same time, the boundary value of the distance between positive samples and negative samples in formula (2) is set to 3. A two-layer GCN is used, that is, in formula (3) is set to 2, and the graph structure embedding dimension learned by GCN is set to 200. The weight parameter in formula (4) is set to 0.2. In the interaction unit, set the maximum number of neighbors of the entity to 50. The number of Gaussian kernels in formula (6) is set to 20, the position parameter in the Gaussian kernel function is set in the range of 0.025 to 0.975, the interval is 0.05, and there are 20 in total. At the same time, set the range of control radial action to 0.1.

4.3 Experimental Results and Analysis

Overall Performance of EA in DBP15K Dataset. To verify the performance of the knowledge fusion model BG-INT that introduces graph structure information proposed in this paper in EA, on the DBP15K dataset, we use the BG-INT model to compare with various EA models. The comparison results are as follows shown in Table 4.

Table 4. Comparing the experimental results of each model on the multilingual dataset DBP15K.

Model	DBP15K$_{ZH-EN}$			DBP15K$_{JA-EN}$			DBP15K$_{FR-EN}$		
	HR1	HR10	MRR	HR1	HR10	MRR	HR1	HR10	MRR
MTransE *[a] [3]	0.308	0.614	0.364	0.279	0.575	0.349	0.244	0.556	0.335
BootEA * [15]	0.629	0.848	0.703	0.622	0.854	0.701	0.653	0.874	0.731
TransEdge [18]	0.735	0.919	0.801	0.719	0.932	0.795	0.710	0.941	0.796
RDGCN [10]	0.708	0.846	0.746	0.767	0.895	0.812	0.886	0.957	0.911
HMAN [8]	0.871	0.987	–	0.935	**0.994**	–	0.973	0.998	–
DGMC [19]	0.772	0.897	–	0.774	0.907	–	0.891	0.967	–
BERT-INT [17]	0.961	0.986	0.971	0.965	0.986	0.974	0.992	0.997	0.994
CEA [13]	0.795	–	–	0.860	–	–	0.964	–	–
SSP [11]	0.739	0.925	0.808	0.721	0.935	0.800	0.739	0.947	0.818
NMN [12]	0.733	0.869	–	0.785	0.912	–	0.902	0.967	–
DINGAL [14]	0.857	0.958	–	0.894	0.973	–	0.971	0.999	–
BG-INT	**0.967**	**0.988**	**0.976**	**0.969**	0.989	**0.977**	0.992	**0.998**	**0.995**

[a]The results of *-marked methods are obtained from [18]. The rest are from their original papers.

The experimental results show that compared with the traditional representation learning model MTransE, the performance of the deep learning model is more advantageous, and various evaluation indicators have been improved a lot. The BootEA model adopts an embedding-based EA self-expansion method to iteratively label possible EAs as the training set, which is a key technique to improve alignment performance. This method outperforms some traditional EA models based on embeddings, compared with For MTransE, HR is increased by about 24% to 30%, and MRR is increased by 30%. For GCN and DGMC using graph structure information, the DGMC model pays more attention to the influence of different neighbor entities on the head entity, so the DGMC model performs better than the original GCN model, with HR1 reaching 77.2%. Compared with the GCN model and the DGMC model, the HMAN model and the BERT-INT model using the BERT model for embedding description are significantly better than other methods and achieve good performance. However, the BERT-INT model uses boundary information, which is different from other models in that this model does not directly aggregate neighbor information, but calculates the interaction between neighbors and captures the fine-grained matching of neighbors. This model is more efficient than some existing models. to have higher performance. The BG-INT model proposed in this paper adds graph structure information on the basis of retaining the interaction modes such as name, description and neighbors. On the public dataset, HR1 has an improvement of about 0.3%.

To further explore the impact of interaction modules on performance in a graph-structured knowledge fusion model, a series of ablation experiments are conducted, and the results are shown in the following Table 5. From the results in Table 5, it can be seen that the maximum pooling operation and column aggregation in the interaction module are deleted, and each index has dropped by about 2%, which can illustrate the importance of the interaction module to the model, delete the neighbor and attribute information, It also makes various indicators drop significantly, indicating that neighbor and attribute information also provides a positive effect on the accuracy of knowledge fusion.

Table 5. BG-INT model ablation experiment results.

Model	DBP15K$_{ZH-EN}$			DBP15K$_{JA-EN}$			DBP15K$_{FR-EN}$		
	HR1	HR10	MRR	HR1	HR10	MRR	HR1	HR10	MRR
BG-INT	**0.967**	**0.988**	**0.976**	**0.969**	**0.989**	**0.977**	**0.992**	**0.998**	**0.995**
Remove components									
-MP	0.835	0.969	0.885	0.864	0.974	0.906	0.968	0.996	0.979
-CA	0.959	0.988	0.971	0.964	0.988	0.974	0.990	0.998	0.994
-N	0.952	0.987	0.965	0.948	0.987	0.963	0.988	0.998	0.992
-A	0.916	0.983	0.942	0.944	0.985	0.961	0.984	0.997	0.990
-N&A[a]	0.835	0.969	0.885	0.864	0.974	0.906	0.968	0.996	0.979

[a]The symbol - indicates deletion. MP means max pooling. CA means column aggregation. N means neighbors. A means attributes. N&A means neighbors&attributes.

Overall performance of EA in CCDataset. The experimental results of the CCDataset are shown in Table 6. It can be seen from the table that although the various indicators of the BG-INT model have decreased compared with the BERT-INT model, the HitRatio@1 of the BG-INT model still reaches 96.5%, which is close to the BERT-INT model, indicating that The BG-INT model still maintains good EA performance in the CCDataset. The reason why the overall performance of the BG-INT model is not as good as the BERT-INT model may be that more than 60% of the entities of the disease type in the CCDataset have less than 15 triples in the two data, making the BG-INT model from entities The learned knowledge about graph structure is insufficient, thus hurting the performance of EA. And in DBP15K, where the number of relational triples is about three times that of CCDataset, BG-INT outperforms BERT-INT, which proves from the side that the graph structure information learned by BG-INT is useful and the entity alignment benefits from the entity embedding that incorporates the graph structure. Meanwhile, we strongly believe that the performance of BG-INT will be further improved in larger public datasets. Finally, after merging the CCDataset according to the EA results of the BG-INT model, 2840 redundant cardiovascular and cerebrovascular data were eliminated.

Table 6. Experimental results of the BG-INT model on the CCDataset.

Model	CCDataset		
	HR1	HR10	MRR
BERT-INT (-attributes)	**0.969**	**0.996**	**0.981**
BG-INT (-attributes)	0.965	0.996	0.978

5 Conclusions

This paper proposes an EA model BG-INT based on BERT and GCN. The model first learns entity name/description, relation and attribute embeddings by fine-tuning the pre-trained model BERT, applies GCNs to learn entity graph structure embeddings, and forms preliminary entity embeddings after weighted concatenation of entity name/description and graph structure embeddings. Then, according to the entity, relationship and attribute embeddings, interaction views are constructed respectively, and the interaction results of each view are spliced to obtain the final entity embedding, to perform EA. Experimental results show that on the multilingual dataset DBP15K, the BG-INT model outperforms the state-of-the-art model by 0.1%–0.6% in HitRatio@1. On the monolingual dataset CCDataset, the HitRatio@1 of the BG-INT model also reaches 96.5%. Finally, after merging the CCDataset according to the EA results of the BG-INT model, 2840 redundant cardiovascular and cerebrovascular data were eliminated.

Acknowledgements. We thank the anonymous reviewers for their constructive comments, and gratefully acknowledge the support of Major Science and Technology Project of Yunnan Province

(202102AA100021), Zhengzhou City Collaborative Innovation Major Projects (20XTZX11020), National Key Research and Development Program (2017YFB1002101), National Natural Science Foundation of China (62006211), Henan Science and Technology Research Project (192102210260), Henan Medicine Science and Technology Research Plan: Provincial and Ministry Co-construction Project (SB201901021), Henan Provincial Key Scientific Research Project of Colleges and Universities (19A520003, 20A520038), The MOE Layout Foundation of Humanities and Social Sciences (Grant No. 20YJA740033), Henan Social Science Planning Project (Grant No. 2019BYY016).

References

1. Auer, S., Bizer, C., Kobilarov, G., Lehmann, J., Cyganiak, R., Ives, Z.: DBpedia: a nucleus for a web of open data. In: Aberer, K., et al. (eds.) ISWC 2007, ASWC 2007. LNCS, vol. 4825, pp. 722–735. Springer, Heidelberg (2007). https://doi.org/10.1007/978-3-540-76298-0_52
2. Xie, R., Liu, Z., Jia, J., Luan, H., Sun, M.: Representation learning of knowledge graphs with entity descriptions. In: Proceedings of the Thirtieth AAAI Conference on Artificial Intelligence, pp. 2659–2665 (2016)
3. Chen, M., Tian, Y., Yang, M., Zaniolo, C.: Multilingual knowledge graph embeddings for cross-lingual knowledge alignment. In: Proceedings of the 26th International Joint Conference on Artificial Intelligence, pp. 1511–1517 (2017)
4. Zhang, Q., Sun, Z., Hu, W., Chen, M., Guo, L., Qu, Y.: Multi-view knowledge graph embedding for entity alignment. In: Proceedings of the Twenty-Eighth International Joint Conference on Artificial Intelligence. International Joint Conferences on Artificial Intelligence (2019)
5. Trisedya, B.D., Qi, J., Zhang, R.: Entity alignment between knowledge graphs using attribute embeddings. In: Proceedings of the AAAI Conference on Artificial Intelligence, pp. 297–304 (2019)
6. Kipf, T.N., Welling, M.: Semi-supervised classification with graph convolutional networks. In: International Conference on Learning Representations (2016)
7. Wang, Z., Lv, Q., Lan, X., Zhang, Y.: Cross-lingual knowledge graph alignment via graph convolutional networks. In: Proceedings of the 2018 Conference on Empirical Methods in Natural Language Processing, pp. 349–357 (2018)
8. Yang, H.-W., Zou, Y., Shi, P., Lu, W., Lin, J., Sun, X.: Aligning cross-lingual entities with multi-aspect information. In: Proceedings of the 2019 Conference on Empirical Methods in Natural Language Processing and the 9th International Joint Conference on Natural Language Processing (EMNLP-IJCNLP), pp. 4431–4441 (2019)
9. Wu, Y., Liu, X., Feng, Y., Wang, Z., Zhao, D.: Jointly learning entity and relation representations for entity alignment. In: Proceedings of the 2019 Conference on Empirical Methods in Natural Language Processing and the 9th International Joint Conference on Natural Language Processing (EMNLP-IJCNLP), pp. 240–249 (2019
10. Wu, Y., Liu, X., Feng, Y., Wang, Z., Yan, R., Zhao, D.: Relation-aware entity alignment for heterogeneous knowledge graphs. In: Proceedings of the Twenty-Eighth International Joint Conference on Artificial Intelligence. International Joint Conferences on Artificial Intelligence (2019)
11. Nie, H., et al.: Global structure and local semantics-preserved embeddings for entity alignment. In: Proceedings of the Twenty-Ninth International Conference on International Joint Conferences on Artificial Intelligence, pp. 3658–3664 (2021)

12. Wu, Y., Liu, X., Feng, Y., Wang, Z., Zhao, D.: Neighborhood matching network for entity alignment. In: Proceedings of the 58th Annual Meeting of the Association for Computational Linguistics, pp. 6477–6487 (2020)

13. Zeng, W., Zhao, X., Tang, J., Lin, X.: Collective entity alignment via adaptive features. In: 2020 IEEE 36th International Conference on Data Engineering (ICDE), pp. 1870–1873. IEEE Computer Society (2020)

14. Yan, Y., Liu, L., Ban, Y., Jing, B., Tong, H.: Dynamic knowledge graph alignment. In: Proceedings of the AAAI Conference on Artificial Intelligence, pp. 4564–4572 (2021)

15. Sun, Z., Hu, W., Zhang, Q., Qu, Y.: Bootstrapping entity alignment with knowledge graph embedding. In: Proceedings of the 27th International Joint Conference on Artificial Intelligence, pp. 4396–4402 (2018)

16. Zhang, K., Ren, X., Zhuang, L., Zan, H., Zhang, W., Sui, Z.: Construction of Chinese medicine knowledge base. In: Liu, M., Kit, C., Qi., Su (eds.) CLSW 2020. LNCS (LNAI), vol. 12278, pp. 665–675. Springer, Cham (2021). https://doi.org/10.1007/978-3-030-81197-6_56

17. Tang, X., Zhang, J., Chen, B., Yang, Y., Chen, H., Li, C.: BERT-INT: a BERT-based interaction model for knowledge graph alignment. In: Proceedings of the Twenty-Ninth International Conference on International Joint Conferences on Artificial Intelligence, pp. 3174–3180 (2021)

18. Sun, Z., Huang, J., Hu, W., Chen, M., Guo, L., Qu, Y.: TransEdge: translating relation-contextualized embeddings for knowledge graphs. In: Ghidini, C., et al. (eds.) ISWC 2019. LNCS, Part I, vol. 11778, pp. 612–629. Springer, Cham (2019). https://doi.org/10.1007/978-3-030-30793-6_35

19. Fey, M., Lenssen, J.E., Morris, C., Masci, J., Kriege, N.M.: Deep graph matching con-sensus. In: International Conference on Learning Representations (2019)

An Semantic Similarity Matching Method for Chinese Medical Question Text

Liru Wang[1], Tongxuan Zhang[2(✉)], Jiewen Tian[1], and Hongfei Lin[3]

[1] Dalian Ocean University of Information Science and Engineering, DaLian 116023, China
[2] Tianjin Normal University, TianJin 300387, China
txzhang@tjnu.edu.cn
[3] Dalian University of Technology, DaLian 116024, China

Abstract. For the purpose of capturing the semantic information accurately and clarifying the user's questioning intention, this paper proposes a novel, ensemble deep architecture BERT-MSBiLSTM-Attentions (BMA) which uses the Bidirectional Encoder Representations from Transformers (BERT), Multi-layer Siamese Bi-directional Long Short Term Memory (MSBiLSTM) and dual attention mechanism (Attentions) in order to solve the current question semantic similarity matching problem in medical automatic question answering system. In the preprocessing part, we first obtain token-level and sentence-level embedding vectors that contain rich semantic representations of complete sentences. The fusion of more accurate and adequate semantic features obtained through Siamese recurrent network and dual attention network can effectively eliminate the effect of poor matching results due to the presence of certain non-canonical texts or the diversity of their expression ambiguities. To evaluate our model, we splice the dataset of Ping An Healthkonnect disease QA transfer learning competition and "public AI star" challenge - COVID-19 similar sentence judgment competition. Experimental results with CC19 dataset show that BMA network achieves significant performance improvements compared to existing methods.

Keywords: BERT · MSBiLSTM · Dual attention network · Text matching

1 Introduction

In the past few years, the data generated in the biomedical field has grown tremendously. With the improvement of living standard and the advancement of science and technology, people are used to searching medical information and obtaining health help on the Internet. At present, automatic question answering system [1] is a popular information access channel in the Chinese medical field, which can provide accurate answers back to users, which can provide simpler and more efficient medical knowledge services for the general public and increase the quizzing experience on the one hand. On the other hand, it can reduce the workload of medical professionals such as doctors and biologists and help improve their work efficiency.

Automatic question answering systems are classified into two types: retrieval and generative, and most medical automated question answering systems are retrieval-based

B. Tang et al. (Eds.): CHIP 2022, CCIS 1772, pp. 82–94, 2023.
https://doi.org/10.1007/978-981-19-9865-2_6

[2]. The Frequently Asked Questions (FAQ) is usually used for frequently asked questions from users, which is constructed by giving a standard question base with one question (Query1) corresponding to one answer. In the process of using, the user's input question (Query2) is matched with the question (Query1) in the standard question base, and the answer corresponding to the question that matches the closest question is returned to the user, so question text matching is the key problem to be solved in medical automatic question answering system. The research on medical question matching algorithm can not only accelerate the development of medical intelligent Q&A, but also accelerate the progress of other fields of natural language processing (NLP) such as recommendation systems, text classification, etc., for exploring the deeper semantic information of the sentences.

Most of the existing works try to use semantic parsing methods [3] to accomplish the matching task, transforming question sentences into semantic expressions such as lambda paradigm [4], DCS-Tree [5], etc. Yao et al. [6] used web-scale corpus matching to extract textual information to accomplish the matching task. Huang et al. [7], Hu et al. [8] and Chen et al. [9] proposed a relevant deep learning algorithm based on NLP can better analyze and process sentences.

In Chinese medical question and answer systems, due to the complexity of medical terminology and the lack of expertise of the questioners, their inability to describe accurately leads to diverse expressions of ambiguities or the existence of textual non-normativity in the question sentences. In order to better understand the semantic information of question text, this paper proposes a pre-trained model based on the siamese recurrent network (Multi-layer Siamese Bi-directional Long Short Term Memory, MSBiLSTM) and a dual attention network to extract deeper text features, and then fuse the obtained token-level features with sentence-level features. The token-level features are then fused with sentence-level features to effectively eliminate the impact on the matching results caused by not considering the real context or by spelling errors or unidentified synonyms, and to optimize the weight distribution by fully considering the importance of the preceding and following sentences to capture the semantic information of the question more efficiently and accurately. The results show that, compared with the model, our model can effectively extract deeper text features from medical question texts, and significantly improve the semantic matching task.

The main contributions of this paper can be summarized as follows:

- We propose to use BERT to obtain two levels of embedding vectors, and fusing token-level and sentence-level feature vectors, as input vectors for the classification layer. In this way, our model feature vectors contain both token-level and sentence-level semantic information, which greatly enriches the semantic representation of the input medical question text.
- The MSBiLSTM is introduced in our model to extract contextual semantic information, which can be well adapted to the irregularities in the medical question text. We also introduce Attentions mechanism to assign weights to the extracted features. The features that play a key role for classification are strengthened and irrelevant features are weakened to further improve the classification effect.
- We experiment on CC19 dataset. The extensive evaluation shows that our method achieves state-of-the-art performance of Chinese medical question matching.

2 Related Work

In order to overcome the shortcomings of traditional search engines that make it diffi-cult to understand user intent and improve the related work efficiency, research related to automatic medical question and answer has attracted increasing attention. In early studies, Athenikos et al. [10] and Jain et al. [11] used rule-based approaches to construct medical question architectures, and Robertson et al. [12] proposed a statistical-based model focusing more on textual information. Heilman et al. [13] and Wang et al. [14] focused on manual feature design approaches to capture word reordering and syntactic alignment phenomena that it can be well applied to specific tasks or datasets, but is difficult to be used to solve other tasks. Lu et al. [15] and Yao et al. [16] used a shallow machine learning approach that can be better self-optimized, but requires a manually designed feature extractor to complete its textual feature representation.

Traditional rule-based or statistical approaches suffer from over-reliance on rule formulation and do not scale easily, or fail to extract deep semantic information from text. With the widespread application of neural networks in NLP tasks, researchers gradually started to explore deep neural network-based approaches. Tan et al. [17] applied a long short-term memory network to obtain information from question text. Thyagarajan et al. [18] and Neculoiu et al. [19] proposed siamese networks to construct models by two LSTMs and compute sentences with Manhattan distance metric of similarity. Wang et al. [20] modeled text matching from different directions and granularity, using four different matching strategies, comparing each time step of the question with the other time steps of the answer. Ming et al. [21] proposed an attention-based model, which uses the representation vector of the question as a memory vector to accomplish text matching. Jing et al. [22] proposed to obtain the sentence by training word vectors and inferring the similarity of sentence pairs based on inter-word similarity. Chen et al. [23] applied a combined model of Bi-directional Long Short Term Memory (BiLSTM) and attention mechanism, which enabled deep interaction between two sentences and formed local inference information to improve the matching accuracy. Cai et al. [24] proposed CNN-LSTM combined with attention mechanism to complete text matching and applied unsupervised clustering method to medical Q&A system to mine users' intention classification. Hong et al. [25] combine siamese CNN structure and translated language model to compute similarity of medical texts.

However, the above methods generally use only a single embedding method or attention mechanism, which will affect the extraction of information obtained from question pairs, while not paying attention to the semantic features of the text context. Moreover, the existence of non-normative or irrelevant text, etc. in the questions asked by medical auto-quiz users will lead to poor semantic matching. To address this problem, this paper designs and proposes a BMA model, which further enhances the model's ability to extract deeper semantic information from Chinese medical question text.

3 Model

In this section, we first offer a general overview of our proposed BMA networks, and then decompose and introduce each component in detail.

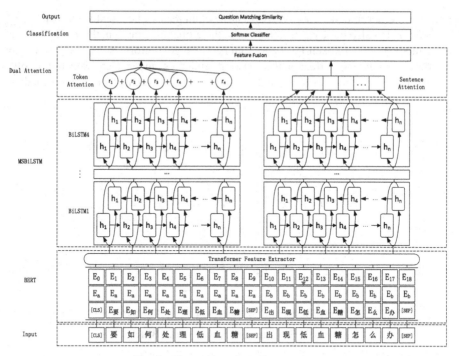

Fig. 1. The architecture of BMA model

The architecture of BMA is shown in Fig. 1. The beginning and end of the question text are represented by [cls] and [sep] respectively as input to the BERT layer, and the three vectors that have been encoded sequences are fused to obtain an adequate vector representation. Feature extraction is completed by a bidirectional Transformer, and token-level and sentence-level feature vector representations are output. The obtained vectors containing rich token-level and sentence-level vectors are input to the MSBiLSTM layer to mine more complex feature representations. Then input to the dual attention mechanism to optimize the weights of important words and sentences, fuse the two feature vectors and input to the classification layer to output the matching degree.

3.1 BERT

BERT [26] is a pre-trained deep language representation model proposed by Google in 2018. Figure 2 presents the Structural framework of BERT. The input layer consists of word, segmentation and location vectors. Its encoding layer is a stack of multiple bidirectional Transformer encoders, and the core is a self-attention mechanism, which can adjust the weight coefficient matrix to obtain the corresponding semantic representation by the word association degree in the sentence.

Traditional word embedding methods mainly focus on the role of words in the global context, lacking the attention to the semantics of the complete sentence, which can lead to the model's inadequate extraction of semantic features of the complete question sentence. Considering that the same token may express different meanings in different problem contexts, in order to make the model not only obtain the local contextual association of the problem, but also increase the attention to the global information, this paper uses the BERT model to obtain token-level and sentence-level text information. This will have a positive complementary effect on the question semantics, and also can effectively solve the problem of accurate word separation and weight assignment in Chinese medical texts, thus improving the semantic matching effect.

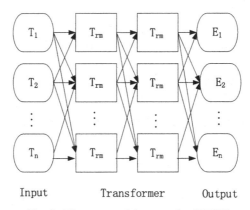

Fig. 2. The structural framework of BERT

In medical question texts, the structure of disease or drug names is generally more complex, for example, they will be combined by multiple letters, numbers, and symbols. Therefore, the three vectors of BERT input layer will play a relatively important role in the medical question matching task. In summary, the BERT model is introduced into our question sentence matching model framework.

3.2 Siamese Recurrent Network

Siamese networks are suitable for finding similarity or a relationship between two comparable things [27]. It is mostly used to accomplish sentence matching tasks and its structure is characterized by the sharing of parameter weights in the sub-networks. Therefore, it does not require too many training parameters, and can solve the overfitting problem. Neculoiu et al. [19] proposed a character-level 4-layer siamese BiLSTM. The embedding matrix is fed into the siamese four-layer BiLSTM. Each step of each layer is forward-backward spliced as the output of that step and sent to the next layer to finally output the vector of each time step as shown in Fig. 3.

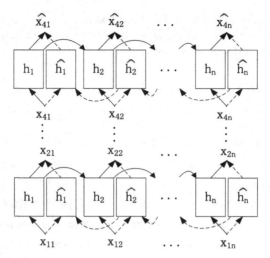

Fig. 3. The structural framework of Four Layer BiLSTM

For each time step the specific computation is as follows:

$$h = g(W_h[h_{pre}, x] + b_h) \tag{1}$$

$$\hat{h} = g(\widehat{W}_h[\hat{h}_{next}, x] + \hat{b}_h) \tag{2}$$

$$x_h = [h; \hat{h}] \tag{3}$$

where g is the logistic function; h_{pre} is the activation vector of the previous memory cell of the forward sequence; W_h, b_h are computed the weight matrix and deviation vector of the computed h respectively; $\hat{h}_{next}$ is the activation vector of the next memory cell of the reverse sequence; $\widehat{W}_h$, $\hat{b}_h$ are computed the weight matrix and deviation vector of the $\hat{h}$ respectively; x_h denotes the output of a layer of BiLSTM and x denotes the input of each time step.

In the actual question, some overly colloquial sentences were found, such as misspelled words and multiple words, as shown in Table 1.

Confusion of Typing and Spelling. In sentence pair Q1, the word " 是" was typed as "shi" in phonetic transcription, which is a common phonetic substitution case.

Synonym Substitution. In sentence pair Q2, "urine sugar $+ + + +$" and "high urine sugar " are common near-synonyms case.

Extra Character. In sentence pair Q3, the letter "B" is added after "diabetes", which is a common multi-character case.

Spelling Mistakes. In sentence pair Q4, the word " 性" is written as " 行", which is a common spelling mistake case.

MSBiLSTM can better adapt to the above text irregularities and extract complex text features more efficiently after the above data extensions. Therefore, we introduce MSBiLSTM into the BMA model framework.

Table 1. Non-normative medical question text examples

id	category	query1	query2
Q1		请问血糖高一点　(6.50)是糖尿病吗	请问血糖高一点　(6.50)sh 糖尿病吗
	Diabetes	Is a high blood sugar level (6.50) diabetes?	Is a high blood sugar (6.50) diabetes?
Q2		为何会出现尿糖　++++的现象	尿糖高的现象是什么原因引起的
	Diabetes	Why the phenomenon of urine sugar+++ appears?	What causes the phenomenon of high urine sugar?
Q3	Diabetes	i型糖尿病怎么治疗	1型糖尿病 B怎么治
		How to treat type i diabetes?	How to treat type 1 diabetesB?
Q4	Asthma	过敏性哮喘应该怎么治	过敏行哮喘应该怎么治
		How to treat allergic asthma?	How to treat allergic asthma?

3.3 Dual Attention Mechanism

The feature words in the question text of the medical auto-quiz play different roles relative to the semantic representation of the complete sentence. In order to reduce the weight of the lesser roles among them, token-level attention is introduced to extract the words that are relatively important to the meaning of the sentence, and the specific computational process is as follows.

$$u_{ir} = tan\,h(W_w x_{hir} + b_w) \tag{4}$$

$$\alpha_{ir} = \frac{exp(u_{ir}^T u_w)}{\sum_r exp(u_{ir}^T u_w)} \tag{5}$$

$$s_i = \sum_i \alpha_{ir} x_{hir} \tag{6}$$

where r is represented as a position in i sentences; x_{hir} is the output of the MSBiLSTM; u_{ir} is the implicit representation obtained by feeding x_{hir} into the perceptron; α_{ir} is the normalized weight coefficient after processing by softmax function; u_w is a random initialization function.

For some sentences with invalid components, such as "Is it good for hypertension patients to drink celery and honey juice in the morning on an empty stomach? Please give a suggestion quickly". It can be seen that the first half of the sentence can indicate the main intention of the question, which should be assigned a higher weight to the first half of the sentence, while the second half of the sentence does not make too much contribution. Therefore, Sentence-level attention is introduced, and the importance of the preceding and following sentences is expressed by a sentence-level context vector, similar to token-level attention, calculated as follows.

$$u_i = \tan h(W_s x_{hi} + b_s) \tag{7}$$

$$\alpha_i = \frac{exp(u_i^T u_s)}{\sum_i exp(u_i^T u_s)} \tag{8}$$

$$v = \sum_i \alpha_i x_{hi} \tag{9}$$

Splicing the above token-level and sentence-level semantic feature encoding results, the adequate semantic feature vector representation of the question text is obtained and calculated as follows.

$$V_p = [s_i, v] \tag{10}$$

Compared with introducing only single-level attention mechanism to optimize the weight distribution and thus improve the accuracy of semantic matching. Therefore, we introduce Attentions into the BMA model framework.

3.4 Clssification Layer

The fused token-level and sentence-level level feature vectors with rich semantic information are input to the classification layer, where the text similarity representation vector is further encoded to learn text matching features effectively. Then the Softmax function is used to feature transform the matching features into a similarity value representation between (0, 1), which is input to the output layer to complete the output of the semantic matching degree of the question sentence. The cross-entropy loss is used as the classification loss of the model, and the calculation formula is as follows.

$$Loss = -\frac{1}{N} \sum_j y_j p_j + (1 - y_j)(1 - p_j) \tag{11}$$

where y_j denotes the true label of the question text pair and p_j denotes the probability of predicting the outcome of the question text pair as a match.

4 Experiments

4.1 Dataset

In this paper, we use the public dataset, referred to as CC19 dataset, constructed by fusing the Ping An Healthkonnect disease QA transfer learning competition and "public AI star" challenge - COVID-19 similar sentence judgment competition, and considering that the dataset contains some repetitive or non-factual descriptions of question sentences, after removing and denoising the invalid data in the experiment, there are 28748 question sentence training pairs and 5749 test pairs, involving 13 disease categories.

4.2 Evaluation Metrics

We calculate the Precision (P), Recall (R) and F1-score (F1) to evaluate the performance of our model. The formula is as follows:

$$P = \frac{T_P}{T_P + F_P} \tag{12}$$

$$R = \frac{T_P}{T_P + F_n} \tag{13}$$

$$F1 = \frac{2P * R}{P + R} \tag{14}$$

where TP indicates the number of matched question texts that are relevant; FP indicates the number of matched question texts that are not relevant; Fn indicates the number of unmatched question texts that are relevant.

4.3 Results and Analysis

To verify the text matching ability of the BMA model, we select several mainstream models for comparison, including CNN-based network models, siamese network architecture-based models, long- and short-term memory-based network models, and network models with an attention mechanism.

The experimental results are shown in Table 2. ABCNN [28] uses two weight-sharing CNN networks, and an attention mechanism is introduced before and after convolution, and the correlation between sentences is considered to construct a sentence model that contains contextual relationships. MuLSTM [29] combines multiplicative LSTM with siamese structures, this architecture learns to project the word embedding of each sentence into a fixed dimensional embedding space to represent this sentence semantics, using cosine to compute the similarity. Fasttext [30] uses n-gram features instead of individual word features, it can achieve similar accuracy as some deep networks on shallow training and can complete text classification more quickly. ESIM [9] uses a two-layer LSTM and attention mechanism, as text enhancement, for splicing and subtraction of long and short-term memory encoding and attention representation. BIMPM [20] uses BiLSTM to complete the encoding of sentence pair embedding in order to make full use of contextual information, and then combines four multi-angle matching operations to complete text semantic matching. STMT [31] computes sentence similarity using a Siamese network structure with BiLSTM and multi-head attention interactions, and enhances model performance with a migration learning strategy. IMAF [32] uses siamese networks to fuse multi-perspective features for multi-layer interaction of textual and structural information to enrich its model feature representation.

The results in Table 2 show that the performance of our model is improved by a large margin, in which our model achieves the highest F1. Compared with the latest model [32], our model does not use a single embedding approach and a single-level attention mechanism. The feature vector contains semantic information at token and sentence levels, which greatly enriches the semantic representation of the input text. For these two levels of feature vectors, MSBiLSTM is used to learn the sequence information

Table 2. Comparison of experimental results of each model (%)

Model	P	R	F1
ABCNN [28]	76.65	75.28	75.96
MuLSTM [29]	77.23	77.87	77.55
FastText [30]	81.60	79.91	80.75
ESIM [9]	83.88	82.61	83.24
BIMPM [20]	87.85	87.66	87.62
STMT [31]	88.23	90.87	89.53
IMAF [32]	88.39	89.43	88.91
BMA	**91.61**	**92.55**	**92.08**

in sentences and words respectively, which is used to extract the semantic information of the context and at the same time can effectively cope with the problems such as text irregularity. The dual attention mechanism in the model assigns the corresponding weights to the obtained features. It will effectively influence the ability of the model to obtain deeper semantic information of the question text, thus improving the matching effect of the semantics of Chinese medical question sentences.

To verify the effectiveness of the MSBiLSTM on the question matching effect in the medical question answering system. Under the condition of using Attentions, we conduct three groups of experiments: without the addition of long and short-term memory, with only the addition of BiLSTM and with the addition of MSBiLSTM, and the experimental results are shown in Table 3.

Table 3. Matching results of different LSTMs (%)

Model	P	R	F1
BERT-Att(s)	86.95	86.47	86.71
BERT-BiLSTM-Att(s)	87.63	91.46	88.02
BMA	**91.61**	**92.55**	**92.08**

From Table 3, it can be seen that there is some improvement in the experimental results using only single-layer BiLSTM, with a precision of 87.63%, a recall of 91.46%, and a F1-score of 88.02%. The analysis shows that the semantic information of the question text can be effectively extracted by adding BiLSTM. And when MSBiLSTM is added, the semantic matching effect is significantly improved compared with the experimental results using only single-layer bidirectional LSTM. Each evaluation index is improved by 3.98%, 1.09% and 4.06% respectively. It is because MSBiLSTM can obtain deeper and more complex semantic information of the question text, effectively eliminating the negative impact of spelling errors and unrecognized synonyms on the matching results, and thus improving the Chinese medical question text matching.

Meanwhile, the experimental results without adding any bidirectional LSTM can be used as ablation experiments for the BMA model, effectively justifying the existence of the MSBiLSTM module in the fusion model structure.

To verify the effectiveness of the Atentions in the medical question semantic matching task. Under the condition of using MSBiLSTM, we conduct three groups of experiments: no attention mechanism added, only token-level attention mechanism added, and Attentions added. The experimental results are shown in Table 4.

Table 4. Matching results of different attention network (%)

Model	P	R	F1
BERT-MSBiLSTM	86.69	86.32	86.50
BERT-MSBiLSTM-Att	87.65	91.04	87.99
BMA	**91.61**	**92.55**	**92.08**

The experimental results show that adding only token-level attention mechanism has improved the experimental results with 87.65% precision, 91.04% recall, and 87.99% F1-score. The analysis shows that the weight assignment can be effectively optimized by adding token-level attention. When the Attentions are introduced, the semantic matching effect is significantly improved, and the evaluation indexes are improved by 3.39%, 1.51% and 4.09% respectively. This is because the introduction of the dual-attention mechanism strengthens the features that play a key role in the question sentences and weakens the irrelevant features, which has stronger representational power in the text comprehension of the question sentences than the introduction of token-level attention mechanism. Meanwhile, the experimental results without adding any attention mechanism can be used as the ablation experiment of the BMA model, which effectively justifies the existence of Attentions mechanism module in the fusion model structure. In summary, it shows that our model can efficiently capture the semantic information of question text and is feasible for semantic matching of medical question text.

5   Discussion and Conclusions

In this paper, we propose a new network for medical question text matching, namely BMA. For retrieval-based medical automatic question answering systems, the BMA model can capture semantic information more efficiently, clarify question intent, and improve question matching. The BERT model is pre-trained to obtain two types of feature vectors, token-level and sentence-level, which can capture more adequate local and global semantic features in the question text. And MSBiLSTM is used to obtain deeper and more complex semantic information, which can make the model better adapted to the phenomena such as text irregularity compared with the basic BiLSTM. Then combine with the dual attention mechanism to optimize the weight assignment, further extract rich semantic features for vector output and fusion, and then improve the accuracy of semantic matching of question sentences. Compared with the existing models, BMA achieves significant performance in medical question text matching. Although our model achieved the best performance on the CC19 dataset, there is still room to improve. The presence of some confusing drug names in the question will lead to a poor semantic matching, for example, "compound paracetamol maleate" and "compound aminophenol bromine" are the same in that they can both be used to treat colds, but different in that They have different ingredients and effects. The current model does not perform well in this problem, so we need to explore the data storage and classification matching of question answer selection in the future.

References

1. Li, T., Yu, H., Zhu, X., et al.: A Chinese question answering system for specific domain. In: International Conference on Web-Age Information Management (2014)
2. Sarrouti, M., Said, O.: SemBioNLQA: a semantic biomedical question answering system for retrieving exact and ideal answers to natural language questions. Artif. Intell. Med. **102**, 101767.1–101767.16 (2020)
3. Berant, J., Chou, A., Frostig, R., et al.: Semantic parsing on freebase from question-answer pairs. In: Proceedings of the 2013 Conference on Empirical Methods in Natural Language Processing. Stroudsburg, PA, USA, pp. 1533–1544. Association for Computational Linguistics (2013)
4. Kwiatkowski, T., Zettlemoyer, L.S., Goldwater, S., et al.: Lexical generalization in CCG grammar induction for semantic parsing. In: Conference on Empirical Methods in Natural Language Processing Association for Computational Linguistics (2011)
5. Liang, P., Jordan, M.I., Dan, K.: Learning dependency-based compositional semantics. Comput. Linguist. **39**(2), 389–446 (2013)
6. Yao, X., Durme, B.V.: Information extraction over structured data: question answering with freebase. In: Meeting of the Association for Computational Linguistics (2014)
7. Huang, P.S., He, X., Gao, J., et al.: Learning deep structured semantic models for web search using clickthrough data. In: ACM International Conference on Conference on Information & Knowledge Management, pp. 2333–2338 (2013)
8. Hu, B., Lu, Z., Li, H., Chen, Q.: Convolutional neural network architectures for matching natural language sentences. Adv. Neural Inf. Process. Syst. **3**, 2042–2050 (2015)
9. Chen, Q., Zhang, X., Ling, Z., et al.: Enhanced LSTM for natural language inference. In: Proceedings of the 55th Annual Meeting of the Association for Computational Linguistics, pp. 1657–1668 (2017)
10. Athenikos, S.J., Han, H., Brooks, A.D.: A framework of a logic based question-answering system for the medical domain (LOQAS-Med). In: Proceedings of the 2009 ACM Symposium on Applied Computing, pp. 847–851. ACM (2009)
11. Jain, S., Dodiya, T.: Rule based architecture for medical question answering system. In: Babu, B.V., et al. (eds.) Proceedings of the Second International Conference on Soft Computing for Problem Solving (SocProS 2012). AISC, vol. 236, pp. 1225–1233. Springer, New Delhi (2014). https://doi.org/10.1007/978-81-322-1602-5_128
12. Robertson, S., Zaragoza, H., Robertson, S., et al.: The probabilistic relevance framework: BM25 and beyond. Found. Trends Inf. Retr. **3**(4), 333–389 (2009)
13. Heilman, M., Smith, N.A.: Tree edit models for recognizing textual entailments, paraphrases, and answers to questions. In: Human Language Technologies: Conference of the North American Chapter of the Association of Computational Linguistics, Proceedings, 2–4 June 2010

14. Wang, Z., Ittycheriah, A.: FAQ-based question answering via word alignment. arXiv preprint arXiv:1507.02628 (2015)

15. Lu, W.: Word sense disambiguation based on dependency constraint knowledge. Clust. Comput. **22**(S3), S7549–S7557 (2019)

16. Yao, X., Durme, B.V., Callison-Burch, C., et al.: Answer extraction as sequence tagging with tree edit distance. In: Proceedings of the 2013 Conference of the North American Chapter of the Association for Computational Linguistics. NAACL, pp. 858–867 (2013)

17. Tan, M., Santos, C.D., Xiang, B., et al.: LSTM-based deep learning models for non-factoid answer selection. Comput. Sci. (2016)

18. Thyagarajan, A.: Siamese recurrent architectures for learning sentence similarity. In: Thirtieth AAAI Conference on Artificial Intelligence. AAAI Press (2016)

19. Neculoiu, P., Versteegh, M., Rotaru, M.: Learning text similarity with Siamese recurrent networks. In: Repl4NLP Workshop at ACL 2016 (2016)

20. Wang, Z., Hamza, W., Florian, R.: Bilateral multi-perspective matching for natural language sentences (2017)

21. Ming, T., Santos, C.D., Bing, X., et al.: Improved representation learning for question answer matching. In: Proceedings of the 54th Annual Meeting of the Association for Computational Linguistics, pp. 464–473 (2016)

22. Jing, W., Man, C., Zhao, Y., et al.: An answer recommendation algorithm for medical community question answering systems. In: 2016 IEEE International Conference on Service Operations and Logistics, and Informatics (SOLI). IEEE (2016)

23. Chen, Q., Zhu, X., Ling, Z., et al.: Enhanced LSTM for natural language inference (2016)

24. Cai, R., Zhu, B., Lei, J., et al.: An CNN-LSTM attention approach to understanding user query intent from online health communities. In: 2017 IEEE International Conference on Data Mining Workshops (ICDMW). IEEE (2017)

25. Cai, H., Yan, C., Yin, A., Zhao, X.: Question recommendation in medical community-based question answering. In: Liu, D., Xie, S., Li, Y., Zhao, D., El-Alfy, ES. (eds.) ICONIP 2017. LNCS, vol. 10638, pp. 228–236. Springer, Cham (2017). https://doi.org/10.1007/978-3-319-70139-4_23

26. Devlin, J., Chang, M.W., Lee, K., et al.: BERT: pre-training of deep bidirectional transformers for language understanding. In: Proceedings of the 2019 Conference of the North American Chapter of the Association for Computational Linguistics: Human Language Technologies, Stroudsburg, PA, pp. 4171–4186. Association for Linguistics (2019)

27. Ranasinghe, T., Orasan, C., Mitkov, R.: Semantic textual similarity with siamese neural networks. In: Recent Advances in Natural Language Processing, pp. 1004–1011 (2019)

28. Pennington, J., Socher, R., Manning, C.: Glove: global vectors for word representation. In: Conference on Empirical Methods in Natural Language Processing (2014)

29. Lv, C., Wang, F., Wang, J., et al.: Siamese multiplicative LSTM for semantic text similarity. In: ACAI 2020: 2020 3rd International Conference on Algorithms, Computing and Artificial Intelligence (2020)

30. Joulin, A., Grave, E., Bojanowski, P., et al.: Bag of tricks for efficient text classification (2017)

31. Wang, K., Yang, B., Xu, G., He, X.: Medical question retrieval based on siamese neural network and transfer learning method. In: Li, G., Yang, J., Gama, J., Natwichai, J., Tong, Y. (eds.) DASFAA 2019. LNCS, vol. 11448. Springer, Cham (2019). https://doi.org/10.1007/978-3-030-18590-9_4

32. Li, G., Liu, X., Ma, Z., et al.: Text matching model incorporating multi-angle features. Comput. Syst. Appl. **31**(7), 158–164 (2022)

A Biomedical Named Entity Recognition Framework with Multi-granularity Prompt Tuning

Zhuoya Liu[1], Tang Chi[1], Peiliang Zhang[2], Xiaoting Wu[3], and Chao Che[1(✉)]

[1] Key Laboratory of Advanced Design and Intelligent Computing, Ministry of Education, Dalian University, Dalian, China
liuzhuoya@s.dlu.edu.com, chitang@s.dlu.edu.cn , chechao@gmail.com
[2] School of Computer Science and Artificial Intelligence, Wuhan University of Technology, Wuhan, China
zhangpl109@whut.edu.cn
[3] Beijing China-Power Information Technology CO., LTD, Beijing, China

Abstract. Deep Learning based Biomedical named entity recognition (BioNER) requires a large number of annotated samples, but annotated medical data is very scarce. To address this challenge, this paper proposes Prompt-BioNER, a BioNER framework using prompt tuning. Specifically, the framework is based on multi-granularity prompt fusion and achieves different levels of feature extraction through masked language model and next sentence prediction pre-trained tasks, which effectively reduces the model's dependence on annotated data. To evaluate the overall performance of Prompt-BioNER, we conduct extensive experiments on 3 datasets. Experimental results demonstrate that BioNER outperforms the the-state-of-the-arts methods, and it can achieve good performance under low resource conditions.

Keywords: Biomedical named entity recognition · Prompt tuning · Low resource

1 Introduction

The biomedical field generates petabytes of clinical data every day, driving the field forward in a number of ways [20]. Medical researchers often have limited ability to analyze data, and they need to use some medical-related processing tools to assist them in analyzing data. The use of deep learning models to extract specific information is the mainstream method in the field of biomedical information extraction at this stage. BioNER aims to extract medically valuable entities such as genes, proteins, diseases, and drugs from unstructured biomedical texts, which provides prerequisites for follow-up work such as relation extraction [2], event extraction [17] and intelligent question answering [8], and also improves the research efficiency of researchers.

© The Author(s), under exclusive license to Springer Nature Singapore Pte Ltd. 2023
B. Tang et al. (Eds.): CHIP 2022, CCIS 1772, pp. 95–105, 2023.
https://doi.org/10.1007/978-981-19-9865-2_7

The explosive growth of biomedical texts provides us with a large amount of unannotated data. Unlike ordinary text annotation, annotation of biomedical text data often requires the participation of professionals, making it difficult to obtain high-quality annotated data [15]. This explains why the volume of datasets in the BioNER domain is usually smaller than that of ordinary the domain datasets. Deep learning models need to be trained with a large amount of annotated data, and the quality and quantity of training data directly affect the performance of the model [22]. This kind of problem restricts the development of BioNER to a certain extent. Using prompt tuning can activate pre-trained model weights with few samples, which can alleviate the problem of insufficient training data for named entity recognition (NER) [16]. At present, few researchers have applied prompt tuning methods to the BioNER task, and even fewer have combined different granularity features based on cue learning.

In this work, we propose a BioNER framework for multi-granularity prompt fusion. Specifically, we construct a prompt-based BioNER main task and an auxiliary task for predicting the number of entities based on prompt learning. By deeply mining biomedical text features at different granularities, a more robust model can be achieved. The work of this paper is summarized as follows:

- We design a multi-task framework based on prompt tuning, which effectively alleviated the impact of the mismatch between upstream and downstream tasks of the pre-trained model.
- We construct an auxiliary task of entity number prediction that introduces supervised signals to mine more implicit features of biomedical texts without requiring additional annotations.
- Experimental results on three few-shot biomedical datasets demonstrate that the proposed framework proposed in this paper achieves excellent performance.

2   Related Work

Fine-tuning pre-trained models is the mainstream approach at this stage. Devlin et al. [5] proposed the BERT model by randomly masking some words of the input utterance and then predicting those masked words. Compared with the previous methods, its effect has been significantly improved. However, BERT and its variants do not perform well in some domain-specific tasks [1]. Lee et al. [10] obtained the BioBERT model on a large-scale biomedical text corpus, as well as achieved good results. Ordinary pre-trained models are very demanding on data, and the insufficient amount of data annotations can lead to a significant decrease in the accuracy of model predictions. Kruengkrai et al. [9] used a framework of multi-task learning to train two models simultaneously with an auxiliary task of manual annotation to obtain more comprehensive information about the text. Tong et al. [21] designed sentence-level and tag-level subtasks based on the BioBERT pre-trained model so that the model captures features with different granularities. Although these tasks have achieved good results, there are still parts that can be improved.

Prompt-tuning methods have become a hot topic recently due to their ability to achieve few-shot named entity recognition. Prompt learning discards the fine-tuning of pre-trained models and uses the method of constructing hint templates to guide the model to predict accurate annotations. Cui et al. [4] proposed a generative named entity recognition model based on BART [11], which uses the decoder structure to predict entity types, and has achieved certain results in the field of few-shot NER. The LightNER proposed by Chen et al. [3] uses a soft prompt approach to reduce the complexity of the model by adding fine-tuneable parameters to the attention part of each layer in the encoder and decoder. Ma et al. [14] proposed the EntLM model, which used the input sentence and the corresponding token-level annotations to obtain more accurate prediction results.

Although methods of prompt learning have made some progress in the field of few-shot named entity recognition, these methods still have deficiencies in the direction of BioNER. What's more, obscure biomedical texts affect the performance of the models. To this end, we try to introduce prompt learning into the field of BioNER and use more implicit multi-granularity features to train the model to improve the performance of the few-shot BioNER model.

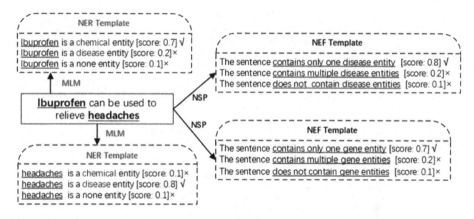

Fig. 1. Prediction example, MLM and NSP represent the masked language model task and next sentence predict task of the BERT pretrained model, respectively.

3   Proposed Framework

The framework proposed in this paper is based on the BERT model and uses the model's original masked language model (MLM) pre-trained task to achieve the BioNER task. In order to make the model perceive features at different granularities, we also construct a new template to implement prompt tuning. It is based on the next sentence prediction (NSP) pre-trained task, which predicts the number of specific entity types in the input utterance. It should be emphasized that in this auxiliary task, we do not introduce additional annotated data, as we can obtain them from the existing NER annotations.

3.1 Main Framework

As shown in Fig. 1, the original sentence "Ibuprofen can be used to relieve headaches" contains two entities, namely, the chemical entity "Ibuprofen" and the disease entity "headaches". We construct a token-level prompt template to predict the entity type corresponding to each word. In addition to this, we construct sentence-level prompt templates for each entity type to predict the number of entities of a specific type in the original sentence.

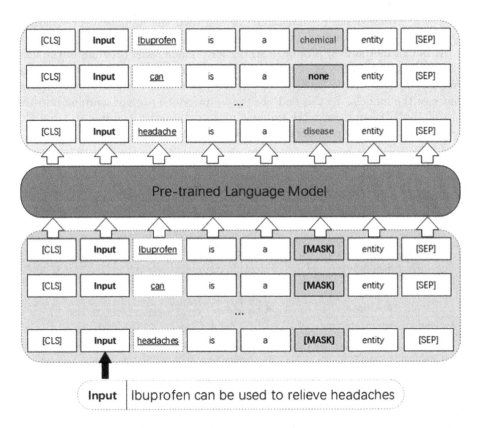

Fig. 2. Example of NER task.

3.2 Named Entity Recognition

As shown in Fig. 2, the named entity recognition work is based on the Mask Language Model task of the BERT pre-trained model. We add the words in the sentence to the sliding window one by one, and finally predict whether the words in the window are specific entities. For the input example "Ibuprofen can be used to relieve headaches", we use "[TOKEN] is a [MASK] entity" as the prompt template. We combine the input sentence and prompt template to predict what entity class [MASK] is using the MLM task of the BERT pre-trained model. This process can be represented by the following formula:

$$P(y|x) = P([MASK] = \mathcal{M}(\mathcal{Y})|x_{prompt}) = Softmax(W_{lm} \cdot h_{[MASK]}) \qquad (1)$$

where $\mathcal{Y}$ denotes all possible entity categories and W_{lm} denotes the parameters of the pretrained model LM head. The predicted words of MASK are selected from a limited class annotation dictionary, which is determined by all entity classes contained in the dataset. For example, the BC5CDR dataset contains two entities, which are a chemical entity and a disease entity respectively, and the entity category prediction word is "chemical", "disease" or "none". To solve the problem that an entity contains multiple words, the size of the sliding window we design can be changed dynamically. In order to prevent the window step size from being too large, resulting in an imbalance of positive and negative samples for prediction, we set the sliding window volume to be less than or equal to four.

3.3   Number of Entities Forecast

Unlike ordinary domains, it is difficult for models to fully understand biomedical entity information if only token-level features are used. Based on the NSP task of the BERT pre-trained model, we construct an entity number prediction template to infer the number of specific types of entities in the input sentence. We construct three hint templates for each entity type, corresponding to the cases where the entity of that type is included in one, more than one, or not included in the original sentence. The original sentences are combined with each prompt template to form the upper and lower sentences input BERT model, and the NSP task is used to predict whether there is an association between the upper and lower sentences, thus realizing the prediction of the number of specific entities. Taking the prediction of disease type entities in Fig. 3 as an example, the input sentence contains a disease type entity "headaches", and then the corresponding prompt template containing a disease type "The sentence contains only one disease entity" is a positive annotation, and the other two prompt templates are negative annotations.

3.4   Model Learning

The NER main task and NEF auxiliary task proposed in this paper extract entity-level and sentence-level features from the text, respectively. The main and auxiliary tasks share the same hidden layer parameters. Without the need for additional annotated data, the model can effectively perceive the type and number of characteristics of entities. We train the model by minimizing the weighted sum of cross-entropy losses for the NER task and the NEF task. The specific formula is as follows:

$$\mathcal{L} = -\alpha \log(p(\widehat{Y}_{NER}|X)) - \beta \log(p(\widehat{Y}_{NEF}|X)) \qquad (2)$$

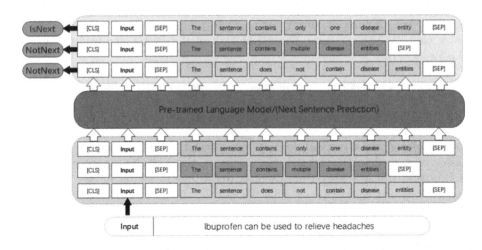

Fig. 3. Example of NEF auxiliary tasks.

Among them, $\widehat{Y}_{NER}$, $\widehat{Y}_{NEF}$ represents the correct label corresponding to the NER and NEF task prediction, respectively, X represents the input sequence. α and β are learnable parameters (hyper-parameters) between 0 and 1.

Table 1. Description of three benchmark datasets.

Dataset	Sentence	Entity type	Evaluation metrics
BC2GM	20,131	Gene or Protein	F1 entity-level
BC5CDR	13,938	Chemical and Disease	F1 entity-level
NCBI-disease	7,287	Disease	F1 entity-level

4   Experiment

4.1   Datasets

Experiments are performed on three public datasets BC2GM [19], BC5CDR [12] and NCBI-disease [6]. The basic information of these three datasets is shown in Table 1. As mentioned in the introduction, we focus on few-shot BioNER work, selecting a small number of samples in the training set of the three datasets to train the model and evaluating the performance of the model on the overall test set. We sample exactly K samples per class for model training and use entity-level F1 values to evaluate model performance, where $K \in \{5, 10, 20, 50\}$.

4.2 Setting

In order to make the framework more suitable for biomedical data, we use Pub-MedBERT [7] pre-trained based on biomedical data as word vector output. We use the AdmaW optimizer [13], with a learning rate set to 5e-5, a valid step size of 1000, and the exponential decay learning rate is adopted.

4.3 Experimental Results

To evaluate the performance of the Prompt-BioNER framework, we compare it with the state-of-the-art models. The baseline models are presented below:

- Single-task model: BiLM-NER [18], a transfer learning model integrating CNN and Bi-LSTM
- Pre-trained models: BioBERT [10] and PubMedBERT [7] pre-trained with biomedical datasets. Here, we conduct comparative experiments by fine-tuning the pretrained model weights.
- Prompt tuning framework: Template-based BART [4], a cue learning framework based on BART [11] pre-trained models.
- Multi-task model: A multi-task learning framework MT-BioNER [21] based on the BioBERT pre-trained model.

Table 2. Performance comparison of Prompt-BioNER and baseline models in three public datasets.

Datesets	Model	5-shot	10-shot	20-shot	50-shot
BC2GM	BiLM-NER	5.60	8.21	18.34	23.87
	BioBERT	14.23	21.53	39.41	58.12
	MT-BioNER	14.41	23.65	39.33	58.92
	PubMedBERT	15.36	22.44	39.67	58.28
	Template-based BART	18.27	25.79	42.72	60.51
	Prompt-BioNER	**19.45**	**26.92**	**43.78**	**61.30**
BC5CDR	BiLM-NER	7.11	12.93	26.90	32.88
	BioBERT	16.04	24.07	43.27	60.35
	MT-BioNER	15.35	25.78	43.34	61.43
	PubMedBERT	16.71	25.03	43.69	60.36
	Template-based BART	20.43	27.22	46.11	62.70
	Prompt-BioNER	**23.13**	**30.10**	**46.64**	**63.24**
NCBI-disease	BiLM-NER	8.60	13.35	25.73	40.01
	BioBERT	16.44	21.90	35.68	63.08
	MT-BioNER	15.87	22.04	35.29	63.34
	PubMedBERT	16.01	21.63	34.52	63.40
	Template-based BART	21.13	24.02	**38.03**	64.54
	Prompt-BioNER	**21.77**	**24.35**	37.54	**65.00**

Table 2 reports the comparative experimental results of Prompt-BioNER and the baseline models. The comparative experimental analysis is as follows:

- It can be seen from Table 2 that compared with PubMedBERT, the overall performance of our method is improved by about 3.9% and 4.3% on the BC2GM and BC5CDR datasets, respectively. This shows that there is a large task gap between the traditional fine-tuning pre-trained models and the upstream and downstream tasks. The impact of the upstream and downstream task mismatch problem is more severe in the case of small samples. The multi-granularity prompt tuning method proposed in this paper enables the downstream task and the pre-trained model to remain largely consistent, achieving excellent performance with low resources.
- The Temple-based BART also uses prompt tuning method. The BART used by Temple-based BART is a pre-trained model based on Seq2Seq. Compared to the PubMedBERT pre-trained model used in this paper, the BART model has an additional Decoder structure and uses more parameters. According to the results in Table 2, our model Temple-based BART was associated with an overall performance improvement of 1.0%, 1.66% and 0.27% on the BC2GM, BC5CDR and NCBI-disease datasets, respectively. This result indicates that the Prompt-BioNER model in this paper can make full use of the pre-trained model weights and uses a reasonable multi-granularity cue learning method to achieve more desirable results.
- Table 2 shows that the performance of all models is improved to varying degrees with the increase of training data. Although the efficiency of improving the F1 value starts to gradually slow down with the increase of training data, our method is still in the leading position under the training data of 5-shot to 50-shot volume. This confirms that our framework is more suitable for BioNER tasks with low resources.

4.4 Ablation Study

To verify the effectiveness of each module, we conduct adequate ablation experiments. In the experiments, we remove specific modules and use different amounts of training data for comparison. The specific experimental results are shown in Table 3.

The results of the ablation experiments in Table 3 show that there is a degradation in the performance of the model after the removal of the entity number prediction task. For example, in the 5-shot experiment on the NCBI-disease dataset, the PubMedBERT framework using the prompt tuning of the NEF auxiliary task obtained an improvement of 1.25 entity-level F1 score. This shows that the NEF auxiliary task can effectively capture the number of entity features in biomedical texts and that such features have a positive effect on the BioNER task.

5   Impact Analysis Between Tasks

In this section, we will analyze the association information between the main task and the auxiliary task.

Table 3. Ablation experiments on three datasets.

Datesets	Model	5-shot	10-shot	20-shot	50-shot
BC2GM	w/o NEF*1	18.45	25.98	42.86	60.51
	w/o NEF*2	18.90	26.00	43.14	60.89
	Ours	**19.45**	**26.92**	**43.78**	**61.30**
BC5CDR	w/o NEF*1	22.56	29.89	46.11	62.42
	w/o NEF*2	23.01	29.56	47.02	62.91
	Ours	**23.13**	**30.10**	**47.64**	**63.24**
NCBI-disease	w/o NEF*1	21.03	24.02	37.51	64.94
	w/o NEF*2	20.52	23.87	37.03	64.47
	Ours	**21.77**	**24.35**	**37.54**	**65.00**

Note: *1 and *2 denote the word vectors output as the underlying word embeddings using the BioBERT pre-trained model and using the PubMedBERT pre-trained model, respectively, both of which are experimented with using the multi-granularity prompt tuning framework proposed in this paper.

In order to more intuitively express the interaction between the main task NER and the auxiliary task NEF, we use 5-shot to 50-shot training data to train the model and select the average F1 score of the test set for comparison to measure the relationship between different tasks. As shown in Fig. 4, on the BC2GM dataset, the NER task brings a 1.80 F1 improvement to the NEF auxiliary task, while the NEF auxiliary task brings a 0.63 F1 improvement to the NER task. The experimental results on the three datasets show that the entity-level NER task is better at mining fine-grained features, and the sentence-level NEF auxiliary task can also bring a certain degree of gain to the NER main task. The two tasks interact with each other and improve the overall performance of the model. In the past, researchers in the field of BioNER focused on entity-level research. A single token-level classification task usually ignores some sentence-level implicit features, such as entity type and quantity features studied

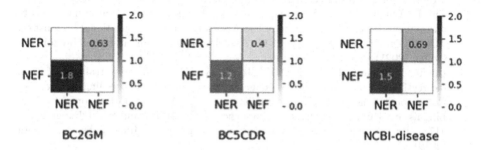

Fig. 4. Experimental results of the main task and auxiliary task on three datasets.

in this paper. However, the training signal brought by this feature can effectively improve the performance of the model on the BioNER task.

6   Conclusion

In this paper, we propose a multi-task approach to prompt learning for the few-shot biomedical entity recognition task, and adapt the traditional sequence annotation approach of the BioNER task to a masked language model task adapted to the pre-trained model, which achieves good results in few-shot biomedical entity recognition tasks. Besides, we create a new auxiliary task of entity number prediction based on the next sentence predict task, which effectively captures the latent features present in biomedical texts. Based on the complementarity of the two tasks, different granularity features are extracted, and finally a robust biomedical named entity recognition model is obtained.

Acknowledgements. This work was supported by the National Natural Science Foundation of China (No. 62076045, 62172074, 61772110), the High-Level Talent Innovation Support Program (Young Science and Technology Star) of Dalian (No. 2021RQ066), Subject of Liaoning Provincial Department of Education (LZ2019002), Program of Introducing Talents of Discipline to Universities (Plan 111) (No. B20070) and Key Program of Liaoning Traditional Chinese Medicine Administration(LNZYXZK201910).

References

1. Beltagy, I., Lo, K., Cohan, A.: SciBERT: a pretrained language model for scientific text. In: Proceedings of the 2019 Conference on Empirical Methods in Natural Language Processing and the 9th International Joint Conference on Natural Language Processing (EMNLP-IJCNLP), pp. 3615–3620. Association for Computational Linguistics, Hong Kong, China (2019)
2. Chen, J., Hu, B., Peng, W., Chen, Q., Tang, B.: Biomedical relation extraction via knowledge-enhanced reading comprehension. BMC Bioinform. **23**(1), 1–19 (2022)
3. Chen, X., et al.: Lightner: a lightweight generative framework with prompt-guided attention for low-resource NER. arXiv preprint arXiv:2109.00720 (2021)
4. Cui, L., Wu, Y., Liu, J., Yang, S., Zhang, Y.: Template-based named entity recognition using BART. In: Findings of the Association for Computational Linguistics: ACL-IJCNLP 2021, pp. 1835–1845. Association for Computational Linguistics, Online (2021)
5. Devlin, J., Chang, M.W., Lee, K., Toutanova, K.: BERT: pre-training of deep bidirectional transformers for language understanding. In: Proceedings of the 2019 Conference of the North American Chapter of the Association for Computational Linguistics: Human Language Technologies, vol. 1 (Long and Short Papers), pp. 4171–4186. Association for Computational Linguistics, Minneapolis, Minnesota (2019)
6. Doğan, R.I., Leaman, R., Lu, Z.: NCBI disease corpus: a resource for disease name recognition and concept normalization. J. Biomed. Inform. **47**, 1–10 (2014)

7. Gu, Y., et al.: Domain-specific language model pretraining for biomedical natural language processing. ACM Trans. Comput. Healthcare **3**(1), 1–23 (2021)
8. Hu, C., Methukupalli, A.R., Zhou, Y., Wu, C., Chen, Y.: Programming language agnostic mining of code and language pairs with sequence labeling based question answering. arXiv preprint arXiv:2203.10744 (2022)
9. Kruengkrai, C., Nguyen, T.H., Aljunied, S.M., Bing, L.: Improving low-resource named entity recognition using joint sentence and token labeling. In: Proceedings of the 58th Annual Meeting of the Association for Computational Linguistics, pp. 5898–5905. Association for Computational Linguistics, Online (2020)
10. Lee, J., et al.: BioBERT: a pre-trained biomedical language representation model for biomedical text mining. Bioinformatics **36**(4), 1234–1240 (2019)
11. Lewis, M., et al.: BART: denoising sequence-to-sequence pre-training for natural language generation, translation, and comprehension. In: Proceedings of the 58th Annual Meeting of the Association for Computational Linguistics, pp. 7871–7880. Association for Computational Linguistics, Online (2020)
12. Li, J., et al.: BioCreative V CDR task corpus: a resource for chemical disease relation extraction. Database **2016**, baw068 (2016)
13. Loshchilov, I., Hutter, F.: Decoupled weight decay regularization. arXiv preprint arXiv:1711.05101 (2017)
14. Ma, R., et al.: Template-free prompt tuning for few-shot NER. In: Proceedings of the 2022 Conference of the North American Chapter of the Association for Computational Linguistics: Human Language Technologies, pp. 5721–5732. Association for Computational Linguistics, Seattle, United States (2022)
15. Moradi, M., Blagec, K., Haberl, F., Samwald, M.: GPT-3 models are poor few-shot learners in the biomedical domain. arXiv preprint arXiv:2109.02555 (2021)
16. Qin, C., Joty, S.: LFPT5: a unified framework for lifelong few-shot language learning based on prompt tuning of T5. arXiv preprint arXiv:2110.07298 (2021)
17. Ramponi, A., van der Goot, R., Lombardo, R., Plank, B.: Biomedical event extraction as sequence labeling. In: Proceedings of the 2020 Conference on Empirical Methods in Natural Language Processing (EMNLP), pp. 5357–5367. Association for Computational Linguistics, Online (2020)
18. Sachan, D.S., Xie, P., Sachan, M., Xing, E.P.: Effective use of bidirectional language modeling for transfer learning in biomedical named entity recognition. In: Machine Learning for Healthcare Conference, pp. 383–402. PMLR (2018)
19. Smith, L., et al.: Overview of biocreative ii gene mention recognition. Genome Biol. **9**(2), 1–19 (2008)
20. Song, B., Li, F., Liu, Y., Zeng, X.: deep learning methods for biomedical named entity recognition: a survey and qualitative comparison. Briefings in Bioinformatics **22**(6), bbab282 (2021)
21. Tong, Y., Chen, Y., Shi, X.: A multi-task approach for improving biomedical named entity recognition by incorporating multi-granularity information. In: Findings of the Association for Computational Linguistics: ACL-IJCNLP 2021, pp. 4804–4813. Association for Computational Linguistics, Online (2021)
22. Zhu, X., Vondrick, C., Fowlkes, C.C., Ramanan, D.: Do we need more training data? Int. J. Comput. Vision **119**(1), 76–92 (2016)

Healthcare Data Mining
and Applications

Automatic Extraction of Genomic Variants for Locating Precision Oncology Clinical Trials

Hui Chen[1], Huyan Xiaoyuan[2], Danqing Hu[3], Huilong Duan[1], and Xudong Lu[1(✉)]

[1] Zhejiang University, Hangzhou 310058, China
lvxd@zju.edu.cn
[2] Chinese PLA General Hospital, Beijing 100853, China
[3] Zhejiang Lab, Hangzhou 311121, China

Abstract. The number of precision oncology clinical trials increases dramatically in the era of precision medicine, and locating precision oncology clinical trials can help researchers, physicians and patients learn about the latest cancer treatment options or participate in such trials. However, unstructured and non-standardized genomic variants embedded in narrative clinical trial documents make it difficult to search for precision oncology clinical trials. This study aims to extract and standardize genomic variants automatically for locating precision oncology clinical trials. Patients with genomic variants, including individual variants and category variants that represent a class of individual variants, are inclued or exclued in accordance with eligibility criteria for precision oncology clinical trials. To extract both individual variants and category variants, we designed 5 classes of entities: *variation, gene, exon, qualifier, negation*, 4 types of relations for composing variants, and 4 types of relations for representing semantics between variants and variants. Further, we developed an information extraction system that had two modules: (1) cascade extraction module based on the pre-trained model BERT, including sentence classification (SC), named entity recognition (NER), and relation classification (RC), and (2) variant normalization module based on rules and dictionaries, including entity normalization (EN), and post-processing (PP). The system was developed and evaluated on eligibility criteria texts of 400 non-small cell lung cancer clinical trials downloaded from ClinicalTrials.gov. The experimental results showed that F1 score of end-to-end extraction is 0.84. The system was further evaluated on additional 50 multi-cancer clinical trial texts and achieved a F1 score of 0.71, which demonstrated the generalizability of our system. In conclusion, we developed an information extraction system for clinical trial genomic variants extraction that is capable of extracting both individual variants and category variants, and experimental results demonstrate that the extracted results have significant potential for locating precision oncology clinical trials.

Keywords: Information extraction · Precision oncology clinical trial · Genomic variant

H. Chen and H. Xiaoyuan—Contribute equally to this work.

1   Introduction

Personalized cancer therapy has shown great promise for improving prognosis for cancer patients, and customizing cancer treatment to a specific genetic profile may improve response and prolong progression-free survival [1]. To confirm the value of a precision cancer treatment for drug development and clinical care, clinical trials prospectively enrolling patients with tumors harboring or lacking genetic alteration X and demonstrating clinical benefit when paired with treatment Y are needed [2]. With advances in tumor biology and decline in the cost of tumor genomic testing [3], there is increasing interest in genomically informed therapy and the proportion of cancer clinical trials requiring a genomic alteration for enrollment has increased substantially over the past several years [4, 5]. The proportion of precision cancer medicine trials compared to the number of all adult interventional cancer trials increased from 3% in 2006 to 16% in 2013 [4] and treatment options in large precision oncology programs changed every 9 months [5]. Researchers, physicians, and patients who want to know about the latest cancer treatment options or participate in such trials need to search for trials on the public registry of clinical trials, such as ClinicalTrials.gov [6]. Despite ClinicalTrials.gov providing partially structured information [7], the genetic variants in clinical trials are still unstructured and non-standardized, so the clinical trials obtained by keyword search are underrepresented and require reading lengthy clinical trial documents to identify potentially relevant trials, making it difficult to quickly and accurately locate precision oncology clinical trials desired to be searched. Much effort has been devoted to developing knowledge bases and search tools to find matching precision oncology clinical trials, such as JAX-CKB [8], OCTANE [9], My Cancer Genome [10], TrialProspector [11], and cBioPortal [12]. However, clinical trials are often curated manually by domain experts in these works, making it a time-consuming and labor-intensive process. This study is intended to automate the extraction of genomic variants from clinical trial eligibility criteria to address an important information need related to personalized cancer therapy.

Genetic variant texts in clinical trials are terms that arise from medical practice and have their own characteristics and complexities. We concluded that genetic variants in clinical trials have the following characteristics, which are why it is difficult to find precision oncology clinical trials. First, the inclusion or exclusion of genetic variants is in the unstructured clinical trial file, and it is not possible to distinguish by keyword search whether the genetic variants are included or excluded in the clinical trial, which means that when searching for a variant you may find some clinical trials excluding patients with the variant. Second, the terminology of genetic variants is ambiguous and hierarchical, and in clinical trials there are not only individual variants but also category variants that represent a category of individual variants, for example, "EGFR mutation" is a category variant that includes all mutations related to EGFR gene. Third, genetic variants are represented in a variety of forms, describing individual variants by {amino acid change, gene} and category variants by {variant type, gene, modifier?, exon?} in most cases. What's more, there are also many genetic variants expressed by distinctive symbols, such as "ALK+", "KRASm+", and "METΔex14". Fourth, there are numerous abbreviations and mergers of genes, exons and amino acid changes, such as "FGFR 1-3", "exon 2, 3 or 4", and "D769H/N/Y".

There have been many attempts to extract genetic variants. Lei et al. [13] reviewed recent advances in automated methods for extracting genomic variants from the biomedical literature, such as MutationFinder [14], tamvar [15], nala [16], and AVADA [17]. These studies extracted genes and variants by rules and machine learning, but they targeted individual variants in the literature, whereas clinical trials have individual variants as well as category variants. Some studies have also attempted to extract genetic variants from clinical trials, for example, Xu et al. [18] defined six different categories of genetic alteration status: GENERAL, WILDTYPE, MUTATION, AMPLIFICATION, DELETION, and FUSION, and detected genetic alteration status by a rule-based system; Zeng et al. [9] designed an oncology clinical trial annotation engine, in which the update module can annotate GENE and MOLECULAR, and thus extracted genomic variants through a lexicon-based approach. These lexicon-based and rule-based methods are not sufficiently generalized to meet the expressive forms of variants arising from the evolving process of tumor biology, and extracting only category variants can bias the extracted genetic variants.

More recently, a novel language representation model, namely Bidirectional Encoder Representations from Transformers (BERT) [19], was proposed by pre-training on large unlabeled corpus using bidirectional transformers [20]. Unlike traditional embedding methods that can only use a fixed vector to represent words with multiple meanings, BERT can dynamically adapt the representation to the context of the words. The pre-trained BERT can be fine-tuned to suit specific tasks such as NER, RC, and Q & A with an additional output layer without significant architectural modifications for specific tasks, and it exhibits more robust performance than traditional CNN and RNN models in biomedical information extraction field [21].

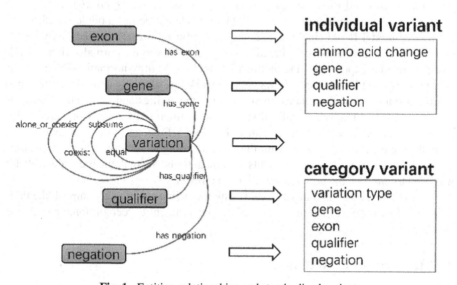

Fig. 1. Entities, relationships and standardized variant

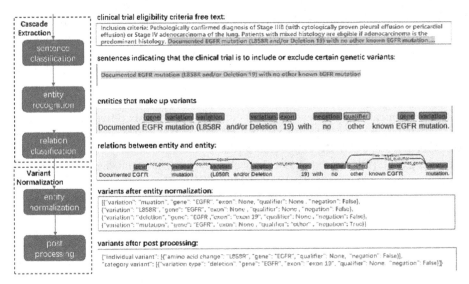

Fig. 2. General workflow of our system

In this study, we developed an information extraction (IE) system to automatically extract genomic variants from clinical trial eligibility criteria. To extract both individual variants and category variants, we designed 5 classes of entities: *variation, gene, exon, qualifier, negation*, 4 types of relations for composing variants: *has_gene, has_exon, has_qulifier, has_negation*, and 4 types of relations for representing the semantics between variants and variants: *equal, subsume, coexist, alone_or_coexist*, as shown in Fig. 1. The IE system had two modules: (1) cascade extraction module based on the pre-trained model BERT, including sentence classification (SC), named entity recognition (NER) and relation classification (RC) and (2) variant normalization module based on regular expressions and dictionaries, including entity normalization (EN) and post-processing (PP). Figure 2 shows general workflow of our system, the system first identified sentences with variants, then extracted the entities and their relationships in the sentences, and finally normalized variants to a structured format. Compared to the previous work, our study features 2 primary highlights. First, the system can extract both individual and category variants with the corresponding annotation scheme depending on the characteristics of genetic variants in clinical trials. Second, the pre-trained BERT was used to improve the generalizability of the model.

We used the pre-trained model BERT, which was fine-tuned to accomplish the three subtasks of cascade extraction: sentence classification, entity recognition, and relation classification.

2 Materials and Methods

2.1 Data and Annotation

We randomly selected 400 non-small cell lung cancer trials from ClinicalTrials.gov. Non-small cell lung cancer clinical trials were used as a validation of our approach because the highest number of precision oncology clinical trials related to non-small cell lung cancer [22]. We extracted the text of eligibility criteria of clinical trials and heuristically divided them into inclusion criteria and exclusion criteria using a rule-based approach, then performed pre-processing, such as splitting sentences and removing unreasonable spaces, and finally randomly selected 400 clinical trials with a total of 800 eligibility criteria texts (400 clinical trials with inclusion criteria and 400 clinical trials with exclusion criteria) for the annotation of genetic variants. It is worth noting that we only labeled genetic variants that were included or excluded in the clinical trials, but not those that were not related to the inclusion or exclusion of genetic variants, such as "drug for EGFR mutation" (Table 1).

Table 1. Definition and examples of entity and relationship

	Category	Definition	Examples
Entity	Variation	Amino acid changes in individual variants, variant types in category variants and genomic variant indicated by special symbols	Del, insertion, T790M, KRASm+, METΔex14
	Gene	The gene in which genomic variants occur	ROS1, anaplastic lymphoma kinase (ALK), FGFR1-3
	Exon	The exon in which genomic variants occur	Exon 19, ex20, exon 19 or 21
	Qualifier	The modifiers describing genomic variants	Activating, sensitivity, germline, somatic
	Negation	The negative word indicating that genomic variant is excluded by clinical trials	Excluded, no, not
Relation	Has_gene	The relation between variation and gene	The relation between "mutations" and "EGFR" in "activating EGFR mutation"
	Has_exon	The relation between variation and exon	The relation between "deletion" and "exon 19" in " exon 19 deletion"
	Has_qualifier	The relation between variation and qualifier	The relation between "mutations" and "activating" in "activating EGFR mutation"
	Has_negation	The relation between variation and negation	The relation between "insertion" and "excluding" in "Evidence of a tumor with one or more EGFR mutations excluding exon 20 insertion."
	Equal	One variant equal or only include another variant	The relation between "mutations" and "deletion" in "Harboring activating mutations of EGFR,only including an exon 19 deletion or an exon 21 point mutation."
	Subsume	One variant include another variant and other variants	The relation between "mutations" and "deletion" in "locally advanced or metastatic NSCLC, with one or more activating EGFR mutations (e.g., G719X, exon 19 deletion, L858R, L861Q)"

(continued)

Table 1. (*continued*)

Category	Definition	Examples
Coexist	Clinical trial include or exclude patients with both variants	The relation between "deletion" and "L858R mutations" in "Subjects harboring both exon 19 deletion and exon 21 L858R mutations are not eligible."
Alone_or_coexist	Clinical trial include or exclude patients with first variant or both variants	The relation between "insertion mutation" and "mutations" in "The EGFR exon 20 insertion mutation can be either alone or in combination with other EGFR or HER2 mutations."

Build on the characteristics of genetic variants in clinical trial eligibility criteria and to simplify the labeling scheme as much as possible to cover most genetic variants, we designed 5 classes of entities: *variation, gene, exon, qualifier,* and *negation*. The definitions are as follows, *variation* is used to label amino acid changes in individual variants, variant types in category variants, and genetic variants indicated by special symbols; *gene* and *exon* are used to label genes and exons in which variants occur; *qualifier* are used to identify modifiers describing variants, such as modifiers describing the nature of the variants; *negation* are used to label negatives indicating the exclusion of a variant. Since these entities are not all proper nouns with specific meanings, their expressive forms and labeling methods are diverse, and we have set up a detailed labeling guideline in order to unify the labeling. Please contact the author to get the guideline if you need it.

We also designed 8 types of relationships. The four relations of *has_gene, has_exon, has_qualifier,* and *has_negation* are the relations that make up variants. To simplify the number of relationships, we consider *variation* as the central entity, and a *variation* entity represents a genomic variant, and the four entities of *gene, exon, qualifier,* and *negation* can be regarded as the attributes of the genomic variant, so that these four relationships composing variants are generated. Another four relations of *equal, subsume, coexist,* and *alone_or_coexist* are used to describe the semantic relationship between variants and variants, *equal* indicates that one variant equals or only includes another variant; *subsume* indicates that one variant includes another variant and maybe other variants, *coexist* indicates that the clinical trial includes or excludes patients with both variants, and *alone_or_coexist* indicates that the clinical trial includes or excludes patients with first variant or both variants. However, due to too few *coexist* and *alone_or_coexist* relations, these two relations were not extracted eventually.

2.2 Cascade Extraction

We used the pre-trained model BERT, which was fine-tuned to accomplish the three subtasks of cascade extraction: sentence classification, entity recognition, and relation classification.

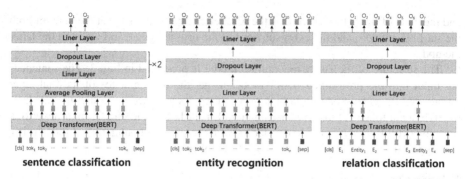

Fig. 3. The model framework

Sentence Classification

To improve the accuracy of variants extraction, the sentences were divided into two categories: positive sentences with a label of 1, which clearly indicate that the clinical trial is to include or exclude certain genetic variants; and negative sentences with a label of 0, which do not contain any genetic variants or do not clearly indicate that certain genetic variants are to be included or excluded. When constructing the training and test datasets, we set the labels of sentences with entities to 1 and those without entities to 0. Owing to the overabundance of negative sentences, 1.5 times the number of negative sentences of positive sentences were sampled randomly. Such sampling would lead to a large number of false positive results, so we predicted the remaining negative sentences that are not in the dataset after one training session, and added the predicted false positive sentences to the training set. The final dataset contains 1561 sentences, of which 1404 sentences are in the training set plus the validation set, and 157 sentences are in the test set.

The structure of the sentence classification model is shown in Fig. 3. The sentences are input into the pre-trained BERT to get the hidden states of its final layer output, and the Average Pooling layer averages the hidden states as the meaning representation of the whole sentence. Finally, the average pooling results are used to predict the sentence labels by the sequential layer consisting of three Linear layers and two Dropout layers that prevent overfitting.

Named Entity Recognition

NER is a basic technique to identify the types and boundaries of entities of interest, and we used NER to identify variant changes, genes, exons, modifiers, and negatives. The sentence tokens were labeled with the BIO tag form, i.e., "B_entity" means a token is in the beginning of an entity, "I_entity" means a token is in the middle or O means that the token does not belong to any entity. So there were a total of 12 tags, with 10 entity-related tags, 1 non-entity 'O' tag, and 1 tag 'X' for the flag bits in the BERT model. It is worth mentioning that since BERT uses the subword algorithm to encode the sentences in order to solve the Out-Of-Vocabulary problem, the word is split into multiple pieces, such as "loved", "loving", "loves" into "lov", "ed", " ing", "es". This results in the token not being able to correspond to the label, so we need to add the corresponding label to the Subword. One way is to set the label of the starting subword as the original label and the label of the extra subword as the X label, another way is to set the label of both the starting subword and the extra subword as the original label, and we used the latter method.

The structure of the entity recognition model is presented in Fig. 3. The sentences are input into the pre-trained BERT model to get the hidden states of its final layer output, and the corresponding hidden states of tokens are used to predict the labels of the individual tokens in the sentences by two Linear layers and one Dropout layer that prevents overfitting. Of course, in order to get the types and boundaries of the entities, we need to further correspond the labels of the token to the entities.

Relation Classification

RE is the task of determining specific semantic relationships between entities, and we used RE to identify the relationships that make up genetic variants and the relationships between variants and variants. Since the number of *coexist* and *alone_or_coexist* relations in the dataset was too small to be used for training, there were a total of 7 relation labels, 4 labels for relations composing variants, 2 labels for relations between variants and variants, and 1 label for negativity. All entity pairs were enumerated in the same sentence, and if the entity type of these entity pairs matched the type of a certain entity pair set by our relations, these entity pairs were added to the dataset; if an entity pair was not labeled, it was labeled with a negative label; if this entity pair was labeled, its label was set to the relation of the entity pair.

The structure of the relationship extraction model is shown in Fig. 3. The sentences are input into the pre-trained BERT model by entity tagging, adding '[unused0]' and '[unused1]' before and after the head entity, and '[unused2]' and '[unused3]' before and after the tail entity, the hidden states of the corresponding tokens of the two entities are stitched together and then input into two linear layers and one Dropout layer to predict the relationship between the entity pair.

2.3   Variant Normalization

Entity Normalization

Due to the large number of abbreviations and shorthand, a labeled entity may contain information about multiple entities, for example, 'VEGF1-2' stands for 'VEGF1' and ' VEGF2'; 'exon 1, 2 or 3' stands for 'exon 1', 'exon 2' and 'exon 3'; 'D769H/N/Y' stands for 'D769H', 'D769N ' and 'D769Y', so the entities were first split based on regular expressions. All the above cases are the splitting of one type of entity into multiple entities of the same type, but a variant change entity may be split into multiple entities of different types. For example, 'del19' is split into *exon* 'exon 19' and *variation* 'deletion'; 'KRASm+' is split into *gene* 'KRAS' and *variation* 'mutation'.

After ensuring that each entity was non-splittable, the entities corresponded to the standard specification. First, we normalized amino acid changes in the *variation* entity and the *exon* entity based on the character rule approach. For normalization of variant types in the *variation* entity, as well as the *gene* and *qualifier* entity, we developed a dictionary lookup procedure, which matchs entities or spelling variations of entities with terms in our dictionaries. Terms for dictionaries were obtained from our annotated corpus as well as from other resources, such as the HUGO Gene Nomenclature Committee [23] and the EntrezGene database [24]. For normalization of the *negation* entity, we specified that whenever *negation* appears or the variant was in the exclusion criteria, the negation was true, and in other cases the negation are false.

Post Processing

Structured variants were obtained based on entities and relationships, and standardized formats for category variants and individual variants were {*variant_type, gene, exon, qualifier, negation*} and {*amino_acid_change, gene, qualifier, negation*}, respectively. These entities that made up the variants were not re-splittable. Remarkably, we removed the tail entity-related variants from the equal relationship because they are duplicated with the head entity-related variants. Furthermore, *variant_type* and *gene* of category variants were non-missable and *amino_acid_change* and *gene* of individual variants were non-missable, so we removed the variants missing these entities. Finally, we removed duplicate and contradictory variants.

2.4 Evaluate Method

To evaluate the performance of a specific task and the overall system, the models were evaluated using three metrics (precision, recall, and F1). For the two tasks of entity recognition and relation extraction, the performance of the model for each entity and relation was also evaluated. To calculate precision, recall, and F1, we first counted T/P/C, where T represents the actual number, P represents the number of predictions, and C represents the number of correct predictions, and then used precision = C/P, recall = C/T, and F1 = 2 * precision * recall/(precision + recall) to obtain the precision, recall, and F1. It is also worth noting that we do not include the negative labels in the calculation, considering that we only focus on the prediction results of positive labels, i.e., the performance of the sentence classification model for non-variant sentences, the performance of the entity recognition model for non-entities, and the performance of the relationship extraction model for entity pairs without relationships were not calculated.

3 Result

3.1 Data Annotation Results

We downloaded 2044 clinical trials about non-small cell lung cancer using the API provided by ClinicalTrials.gov, from which 400 clinical trials with a total of 800 eligibility criteria texts (inclusion criteria for 400 clinical trials and exclusion criteria for 400 clinical trials) were randomly selected for annotation. We split these 400 clinical trials into a training set and a test set in a 7:1 ratio, and descriptive statistics of the annotated corpus are presented in Table 2.

Table 2. Descriptive statistics of the annotated corpus.

Statistics		Training set	Testing set
Number of clinical trials		350	50
Number of clinical triasl with variants		262	41
Number of sentences with variants		479	61
Average word number of sentences with variants		26.68	26.21
Average token number of sentences with variants		40.47	39.69
Entity	Gene	665	87
	Qualifier	213	24
	Variation	991	116
	Exon	206	26
	Negation	64	6
Relation	Has_gene	756	91
	Has_qualifier	212	27
	Has_exon	211	26
	Has_negation	76	12
	Equal	207	12
	Subsume	94	20

3.2 Model Evaluate Results

Cascade Extraction Evaluate Results

For the three subtasks of cascade extraction: SC, NER and RE, we randomly selected a training set with a ratio of 0.15 as the validation set and used an early stopping strategy on the validation set, that is, the model stopped training when the performance on the validation set no longer increased for 10 epochs in a row, so as to achieve the effect of adequate training and avoid overfitting. The model with the best performance on the validation set was selected as the final model and tested in the test set. The evaluation results of the models in the validation and test sets are shown in Table 3, where the F1 of SC, NER and RE, were 0.9709, 0.9353, and 0.9485 in the validation set, and 0.9841, 0.9135, and 0.9509 in the test set, respectively.

The analysis of the prediction results for each subtask reveals that the errors mainly originate from false positives. For SC, the sentences that the model is prone to misidentify are those containing descriptions related to variants, such as "If available, tumor tissue should be submitted for EGFR status by IHC and correlative studies." (NCT00492206), and those with similar formatting to variants, such as "HBsAg positive, HBV DNA $\geq$ 1000 cps/ml (or200IU/ml)." (NCT03787992). For NER, entities that are not proper nouns with specific meanings are also labeled, for example, "sensitizing" is labeled as an entity

Table 3. The result of model evaluation.

Module	Label	Validation set				Test set			
		Precision	Recall	F1	T/P/C	Precision	Recall	F1	T/P/C
Sentence classification	Positive	0.9524	0.9901	0.9709	101/105/100	0.9841	0.9841	0.9841	63/63/62
Entity recognition	Gene	0.9183	0.9474	0.9326	95/98/90	0.8632	0.9425	0.9011	87/95/82
	Variation	0.9685	0.9625	0.9655	160/160/156	0.9417	0.9741	0.9576	116/120/113
	Exon	0.9310	1.0000	0.9643	27/29/27	0.9230	0.9230	0.9230	26/26/24
	Qualifier	0.8250	0.8250	0.8250	40/40/33	0.7692	0.8333	0.8000	24/26/20
	Negation	0.8750	0.7778	0.8235	9/8/7	0.6667	0.6667	0.6667	6/6/4
	All_entity	0.9311	0.9396	0.9353	331/334/311	0.8901	0.9382	0.9135	259/273/243
Relation extraction	Has_gene	0.9580	0.9828	0.9702	116/119/114	0.9474	0.9890	0.9677	91/95/90
	Has_exon	0.9706	0.9429	0.9565	35/34/33	0.9615	0.9615	0.9615	26/26/25
	Has_nagation	1.0000	0.7273	0.8421	11/8/8	0.9167	0.9167	0.9167	12/12/11
	Has_qualifier	1.0000	0.9459	0.9722	37/35/35	0.9630	0.9630	0.9630	27/27/26
	Subsume	0.7500	0.9000	0.8182	10/12/19	1.0000	1.0000	1.0000	20/20/20
	Equal	0.8462	0.9565	0.8980	23/26/22	0.6316	1.0000	0.7742	12/19/12
	All_relation	0.9444	0.9526	0.9485	232/234/221	0.9246	0.9787	0.9509	188/199/184
Standardization						0.9369	0.9720	0.9541	107/111/104
End-to-end evaluate						0.8053	0.8505	0.8273	107/113/91
Ablation experiment						0.6190	0.8505	0.7165	107/147/91
Multi-cancer evaluation						0.6215	0.8313	0.7113	160/214/133

qualifier in "Documentation of a sensitizing mutation of the epidermal growth factor receptor", but many words with the similar meaning may be incorrectly considered as a *qualifier* by the model, such as "sensitivity" in "High likelihood of gefitinib sensitivity" (NCT00372515); in addition, words with similar morphology can also be misidentified, such as "RAD51C/D "(NCT02264678) represents "RAD51C" gene and "RAD51D" gene, but they are incorrectly identified as entity *variation* because they resemble amino acid change in the character structure. For RE, the model can easily learn these patterns because the descriptions in many sentences are similar. However, for some pairs of entities that are far apart, their relationships are easily not recognized; in addition, if the sentence length is too long and the entities and relationships are at the end of the sentence, the model is likely to fail to recognize them.

Variant Normalization Evaluate Results
To evaluate the performance of variant normalization module, the genetic variants were manually organized in the test set in the structured format as our gold standard. Then we input the test set corpus (manually annotated entities and relations) to variant normalization module to obtain the extracted genetic variants. Since the entities and relations were manually annotated, this part was considered reliable, then we compared the extracted genetic variants with the gold standard to get the performance of variant normalization part of the module. We implemented precision matching, which requires variants to be exactly the same as that in the gold standard results. The final evaluation results of the standardization module were 0.9369 for precision, 0.9720 for recall, 0.9541 for F1, and 107/111/104 for T/P/C.

End-to-End Evaluate Results
The evaluation steps in this section were similar to variant normalization, which was also compared with the gold standard, with the difference that instead of using a manually annotated corpus, we extracted the entities and relationships of the variants through the model and obtain the final structured variants. The final model was evaluated to have a precision of 0.8053, a recall of 0.8505, an F1 of 0.8273, and a T/P/C of 107/113/91, indicating that the model was able to extract the majority of genetic variants from the clinical trial eligibility criteria.

To validate the generalizability of our method and model across multiple cancer types, an additional engineer screened 50 clinical trials containing gene variants in unrestricted cancer areas and compiled structured gene variants according to our annotation guidelines and standardized format. This engineer had not previously participated in our annotation and model-building efforts. Comparing the results extracted from our system with it, the evaluation results were 0.6215 for precision, 0.8313 for recall, 0.7113 for F1, and 160/214/133 for T/P/C. This result showed a higher decrease in precision compared to the evaluation results in the NSCLC corpus, which may be due to the model in the new cancer corpus incorrectly identifying sentences or entities associated with gene variants, on the other hand, it may be because the new engineers missed some gene variants during annotation.

4 Discussion

4.1 The Effect of Sentence Classification

A highlight of this study is the use of SC to filter sentences containing descriptions related to gene variants but not clearly indicating that certain genetic variants are to be included or excluded, which avoids many false positive results. The idea originated from the paper [25] that used sentence classification to improve the performance of entity recognition. To verify the role of SC in the model, we conducted ablation experiments. In the cascade extraction module, only NER and RE were used, and SC was no longer used, and the results of the end-to-end ablation experiment were evaluated as 0.6190 for precision, 0.8505 for recall, 0.7165 for F1, and 107/147/91 for T/P/C. Compared with the results of the model using SC, recall was unchanged and precision was reduced. This indicates that SC can filter some false positive results because sentence classification removes sentences that contain genetic variants but do not include or exclude them.

4.2 The Limitations of Our Work

Although the developed system achieves a good overall performance in genetic variant extraction, there are still some limitations of our work.

Firstly, the annotation scheme didn't cover all genetic variants that appear in the eligibility criteria for clinical trials, and some genetic variants that appear less frequently were not annotated, for example, "Ras mutations must be one of the following point mutations at codon 12" (NCT00019331) uses the amino acid position "codon 12" to describe the variant; "Glycine to valine" (NCT00019331) uses natural language to describe amino acid changes. In addition, less frequent relationships were not marked, such as "patients with EML4-ALK translocations". (NCT01124864) where the *gene* "EML4" and *gene* "ALK" should set a fusion relationship, and the *gene* "EGFR" and *exon* "exon 20" in "abnorm of EGFR exon 20, KRAS, BRAF" should have a linkage relationship. Since these entities and relationships were not labeled, extracted variants will be biased.

The imbalance in the number of labeled entities and relations had a great impact on the effectiveness of extraction. Although we labeled *coexist* and *alone_or_coexist* relations, the number of labeling was too small to train. The importance of coexisting variants for patient treatment is being gradually emphasized [26]. Moreover, the extraction effect of the relatively small number of entities and relations was worse compared with the large number of entities and relations, for example, F1 of *negation, qualifier*, and *equal* was only 0.667, 0.800 and 0.774. Possible solutions to this problem are labeling more data and using oversampling for data balancing.

The hierarchical relationship between category variants and individual variants is essential for the retrieval of clinical trials related to genetic variants. The category variant "EGFR activating mutation" includes the category variant "EGFR exon 19 deletion", and the category variant "EGFR exon 19 deletion" includes the individual variant "EGFR L858R", we want to search all clinical trials for "EGFR L858R", it is also necessary to search for "EGFR exon 19 deletion" and "EGFR activating mutation" related clinical trials. An ideal idea is to assign all clinical trials to individual variants, so that we can automatically search directly based on the patient's genetic test results. We use the semantic relations between variants *subsume* and *equal* to obtain the variant hierarchy, but we find that the hierarchy table obtained in this way is limited, and more hierarchies may need to be sorted out manually.

5   Conclusion

In this study, we developed an IE system that automatically extracts information on genetic variants including individual variants and category variants from non-small cell lung cancer clinical trial eligibility criteria. The experimental results show that the IE system can effectively use SC to filter sentences that contain genetic variants but don't include or exclude genetic variants, use NER and RC to extract entities and relationships associated with genetic variants, and use the variant normalization module to obtain structured genetic variants. In addition, this IE system can not only effectively extract genetic variants in non-small cell lung cancer clinical trials, but also achieves good results in genetic variants extraction in multi-cancer clinical trials.

Precision oncology clinical trials targeting genetic variants develop new treatment options for oncology patients, and patients entering clinical trials are likely to receive better and more advanced treatments [27]. Genetic variants we extract can help researchers, physicians, and patients locate precision oncology clinical trials on the one hand and help patients enroll in clinical trials on the other.

Acknowledgements. This work was supported by the National Natural Science Foundation of China [grant numbers 82172070].

References

1. Schwaederle, M., et al.: Association of biomarker-based treatment strategies with response rates and progression-free survival in refractory malignant neoplasms: a meta-analysis. JAMA Oncol. **2**(11), 1452–1459 (2016)
2. Biankin, A.V., Piantadosi, S., Hollingsworth, S.J.: Patient-centric trials for therapeutic development in precision oncology. Nature **526**(7573), 361–370 (2015)
3. Taber, K.A.J., Dickinson, B.D., Wilson, M.: The promise and challenges of next-generation genome sequencing for clinical care. JAMA Intern. Med. **174**(2), 275–280 (2014)
4. Roper, N., Stensland, K.D., Hendricks, R., Galsky, M.D.: The landscape of precision cancer medicine clinical trials in the United States. Cancer Treat. Rev. **41**(5), 385–390 (2015)
5. Araya, A., et al.: Rate of change in investigational treatment options: an analysis of reports from a large precision oncology decision support effort. Int. J. Med. Inform. **143**, 104261 (2020). https://doi.org/10.1016/j.ijmedinf.2020.104261
6. ClinicalTrials.gov: ClinicalTrials.gov (2022). https://clinicaltrials.gov/. Accessed 22 Aug 2022
7. Zarin, D.A., Williams, R.J., Tse, T., Ide, N.C.: The role and importance of clinical trial registries and results databases. Princ. Pract. Clin. Res., 111–125 (2018)
8. Patterson, S.E., Liu, R., Statz, C.M., Durkin, D., Lakshminarayana, A., Mockus, S.M.: The clinical trial landscape in oncology and connectivity of somatic mutational profiles to targeted therapies. Hum. Genomics **10**(1), 1–13 (2016)

9. Zeng, J., et al.: OCTANE: oncology clinical trial annotation engine. JCO Clin. Cancer Inform. (3), 1–11 (2019). https://doi.org/10.1200/CCI.18.00145

10. Micheel, C.M., Lovly, C.M., Levy, M.A.: My cancer genome. Cancer Genet. **207**(6), 289 (2014)

11. Sahoo, S.S., et al.: Trial prospector: matching patients with cancer research studies using an automated and scalable approach. Cancer Inform. **13**, S19454 (2014)

12. Unberath, P., Mahlmeister, L., Reimer, N., Busch, H., Boerries, M., Christoph, J.: Searching of clinical trials made easier in cBioPortal using patients' genetic and clinical profiles. Appl. Clin. Inform. **13**(02), 363–369 (2022)

13. Lee, K., Wei, C., Lu, Z.: Recent advances of automated methods for searching and extracting genomic variant information from biomedical literature. Brief. Bioinform. (2020). https://doi.org/10.1093/bib/bbaa142

14. Caporaso, J.G., Baumgartner, W.A., Jr., Randolph, D.A., Cohen, K.B., Hunter, L.: MutationFinder: a high-performance system for extracting point mutation mentions from text. Bioinformatics **23**(14), 1862–1865 (2007)

15. Wei, C., Phan, L., Feltz, J., Maiti, R., Hefferon, T., Lu, Z.: tmVar 2.0: integrating genomic variant information from literature with dbSNP and ClinVar for precision medicine. Bioinformatics **34**(1), 80–87 (2018). https://doi.org/10.1093/bioinformatics/btx541

16. Cejuela, J.M., et al.: nala: text mining natural language mutation mentions. Bioinformatics **33**(12), 1852–1858 (2017). https://doi.org/10.1093/bioinformatics/btx083

17. Birgmeier, J., et al.: AVADA: toward automated pathogenic variant evidence retrieval directly from the full-text literature. Genet. Med. **22**(2), 362–370 (2020). https://doi.org/10.1038/s41436-019-0643-6

18. Xu, J., et al.: Extracting genetic alteration information for personalized cancer therapy from ClinicalTrials.gov. J. Am. Med. Inform. Assoc. **23**(4), 750–757 (2016). https://doi.org/10.1093/jamia/ocw009

19. Devlin, J., Chang, M., Lee, K., Toutanova, K.: BERT: pre-training of deep bidirectional transformers for language understanding. arXiv preprint arXiv:1810.04805 (2018)

20. Vaswani, A., et al.: Attention is all you need. In: Advances in Neural Information Processing Systems, vol. 30 (2017)

21. Lee, J., et al.: BioBERT: a pre-trained biomedical language representation model for biomedical text mining. Bioinformatics **36**(4), 1234–1240 (2020)

22. Del Paggio, J.C., et al.: Evolution of the randomized clinical trial in the era of precision oncology. JAMA Oncol. **7**(5), 728–734 (2021). https://doi.org/10.1001/jamaoncol.2021.0379

23. Seal, R.L., Gordon, S.M., Lush, M.J., Wright, M.W., Bruford, E.A.: Genenames. org: the HGNC resources in 2011. Nucleic Acids Res. **39**(Suppl._1), D514–D519 (2010)

24. Maglott, D., Ostell, J., Pruitt, K.D., Tatusova, T.: Entrez gene: gene-centered information at NCBI. Nucleic Acids Res. **33**(Suppl._1), D54–D58 (2005)

25. Dhayne, H., Kilany, R., Haque, R., Taher, Y.: EMR2vec: bridging the gap between patient data and clinical trial. Comput. Ind. Eng. **156**, 107236 (2021). https://doi.org/10.1016/j.cie.2021.107236

26. Guo, Y., et al.: Concurrent genetic alterations and other biomarkers predict treatment efficacy of EGFR-TKIs in EGFR-mutant non-small cell lung cancer: a review. Front. Oncol. **10**, 610923 (2020)

27. Ettinger, D.S., et al.: Non–small cell lung cancer, version 3.2022, NCCN clinical practice guidelines in oncology. J. Natl. Compr. Cancer Netw. **20**(5), 497–530 (2022)

Identification of Sepsis Subphenotypes Based on Bi-directional Long Short-Term Memory Auto-encoder Using Real-Time Laboratory Data Collected from Intensive Care Units

Yongsen Tan[1], Jiahui Huang[1], Jinhu Zhuang[1], Haofan Huang[1], Yong Liu[2], and Xiaxia Yu[1(✉)]

[1] School of Biomedical Engineering, Health Science Center, Shenzhen University, Shenzhen, China
xiaxiayu@szu.edu.cn

[2] Department of Intensive Care Unit, Shenzhen Hospital, Southern Medical University, Shenzhen, China

Abstract. Sepsis is a heterogeneous syndrome characterized by a dysregulated immunological response to infection that results in organ dysfunction and often death. Identification of clinically relevant subphenotypes, which could potentially lead to personalized sepsis management. A clustering framework was proposed to identify sepsis subphenotypes using the bidirectional long short-term memory Auto-Encoder (BiLSTM-AE) together with the k-means algorithm. The subphnotypes were determined according to the proposed algorithm. After that, each subphnotype was evaluated according to their inpatient mortality rate. In addition, sensitivity was performed to evaluate the robust of the predictiveness of the model-learned representation and clinical significance. A total of 971 patients with 4905 records meeting the clustering criteria after data processing were included in the study. There were 748 patients (77.0%) with an overall in-hospital mortality rate of 2.9% in subphenotype 1, 120 (12.4%) with 10.0% mortality rate in subphenotype 2, and 103 (10.6%) with 78.6% mortality rate in subphenotype 3. Some laboratory biomarkers showed significant differences between different sepsis subphenotypes, such as AST (subphenotype 1: 61.0 vs. subphenotype 2: 75.5 vs. subphenotype 3: 298.6, units/L; $P < 0.001$) and ALT (subphenotype 1: 49.8 vs. subphenotype 2: 59.3 vs. subphenotype 3: 200.2, units/L; $P < 0.001$). The area under the receiver operating characteristic curve (AUROC) in this study was 0.89, and the area under precision recall curve (AUPRC) was 0.65. In this study, sepsis subphenotypes were identified using clustering framework based on BiLSTM-AE and k-means. This research may drive the personalization of sepsis management and provide new insights and guidance for subphenotype research.

Keywords: Sepsis subphenotypes · Time series · BiLSTM-AE · Clustering

---

Y. Tan and J. Huang—These authors contributed equally to this work.

B. Tang et al. (Eds.): CHIP 2022, CCIS 1772, pp. 124–134, 2023.
https://doi.org/10.1007/978-981-19-9865-2_9

1 Background

Sepsis is a systemic inflammatory response to infection that involves humoral and cellular responses, as well as circulatory abnormalities [1, 2]. Importantly, sepsis is a heterogeneous clinical syndrome that is the leading cause of mortality in hospital intensive care units [3]. Treating a septic patient is highly challenging because individual patients respond differently to medical interventions. Identification of sepsis subphenotypes may lead to more precise treatments and more targeted clinical interventions.

Over the past few decades, there have been many studies on patients in hospital intensive care units (ICUs) using electronic health records (EHRs) [4, 5], but only a few studies have tried identification of sepsis subphenotypes based on the variables' temporality. Bhanvani et al. performed temperature trajectory modeling to identify subtypes [6]. Yin et al. proposed a new sepsis subtyping framework to deal with temporality of EHR data and missing values issues [7]. Most existing studies [8, 9] have used traditional methods such as latent class analysis (LCA) to identify subphenotypes which ignores the variables' temporality, an important characteristic of EHR data.

Notably, in ICU settings, the important data such as laboratory measurements are usually stored densely compared with a normal in-hospital ward in a timely manner. These time series data reflect changes in pathophysiological features of sepsis. Therefore, we proposed a novel architecture depending on deep learning using time series data to identify subphenotypes. The proposed architecture contained two steps. The first was to generate specific representations from the input data using bidirectional long short-term memory Auto-Encoder (BiLSTM-AE), and the second was to identify subphenotypes using these representations and the k-means algorithm. Furthermore, we also evaluated the ability of mortality risk prediction based on this novel sepsis subphenotypes.

2 Methods

2.1 Patient Selection

For this retrospective cohort study, the eICU Collaborative Research Database was used [10]. It is a multicenter ICU database with high granularity data for over 200,000 admissions to ICUs monitored by the eICU Programs across the United States [11]. In this study, all patients were diagnosed with sepsis-3 in the ICU in line with the sepsis definitions revised by the Third International Consensus Definitions for Sepsis and Septic Shock (Sepsis-3) [12]. Therefore, the patients with a SOFA ≥ 2 within 24 h of suspected infection were selected (Fig. 1). Patients who were younger than 18 years or spent less than 24 h in the ICU were excluded.

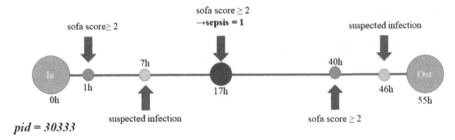

Fig. 1. The diagnostic criteria of sepsis

2.2 The Time Series Input Features and Data Processing

The main objective of the present study was to identify subphenotypes of sepsis patients using the routinely collected data in ICUs. A list of time series data were included: magnesium, mean corpuscular hemoglobin, blood urea nitrogen, lymphocytes, chloride, eosinophilic granulocytes, platelets, mean corpuscular volume, red blood cells, red cell distribution width, mean corpuscular hemoglobin concentration, white blood cells, creatinine, calcium, hemoglobin, bicarbonate, potassium, polymorphonuclear neutrophils, monocytes, total bilirubin, basophilic granulocytes, alanine transaminase, hematocrit, aspartate transaminase, glucose, total protein, sodium, albumin, and bedside glucose as the routinely collected data that are available in almost every patient in the ICU. The values were grouped according to the 24-h interval, and the mean value was derived for each interval. To acquire a more homogeneous population, patients with records for less than 90% of these features were removed.

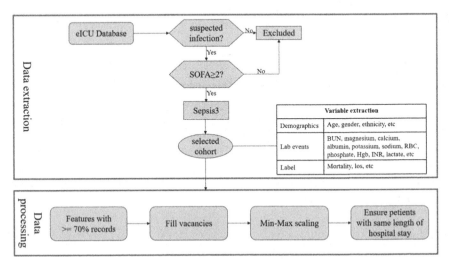

Fig. 2. The workflow for data extraction and processing. Patients diagnosed with sepsis-3 were included. The data processing steps included filtering features, filling vacancies, standardization, and determining the observation window. (BUN, blood urea nitrogen; Hgb, hemoglobin; INR, international normalized ratio; RBC, red blood cells; los, length of ICU stay)

Data processing was then performed and shown in Fig. 2. Records that included over 70% of these features were chosen to avoid significant interference of unrecorded information in the EHR. Then, the mean of each feature was calculated to fill vacancies. Min-Max scaling was conducted on the data to ensure the values were within a particular range. There were different lengths of hospitalization data for each patient. Therefore, 14 days as a time observation window was set to ensure that each patient possessed the same length of hospital stay, which means that hospital records with a lengthy stay were truncated, while zero imputation was used for records with short stays. The time observation window started 24 h after admission.

2.3 Algorithm

Feature Encoding

The first key step for our method was to acquire effective and appropriate representation vectors for all patients. The laboratory measurement of each patient during hospitalization constituted a separate individual table. Therefore, multiple patients with different hospital stays and measurements formed three-dimensional raw time series data.

The overall architecture of our algorithm is shown in Fig. 3. BiLSTM-AE was introduced to perform feature encoding for the input time series data. BiLSTM can improve performance for sequence classification problems compared with the traditional LSTM [13]. LSTM only retains past information, while BiLSTM can save former and future information at any time point [14]. Our network was composed of two parts, the encoder and decoder. The encoder converted the input data to internal representations, and the decoder converted representations to the output for prediction. This was a process of compression and decompression, which could learn high-level representations of input features. The above procedure was data-driven, making the input data and the representation output strongly correlated.

Clustering

After the construction of the representations, the k-means algorithm was used to identify sepsis subphenotypes. The k-means algorithm is a widely used clustering method based on Euclidean distance [15]. It generally requires the value of k to be specified to obtain the number of subphenotypes. The clustering performance with different k values was evaluated using the silhouette coefficient score, which combined two factors, including cohesion and separation. In addition, t-distributed stochastic neighbor embedding (t-SNE) was used to visualize the clustering result [16].

Mortality Prediction

A predictor was constructed for mortality prediction in this step. The predictor consisted of three parts, including two different linear layers and a Softmax layer. The representations obtained from the previous step were input into the predictor, and then it was trained to obtain the predicting mortality probability. The binary cross entropy (BCE) loss was used to constrain the parameter weights to acquire more accurate prediction values.

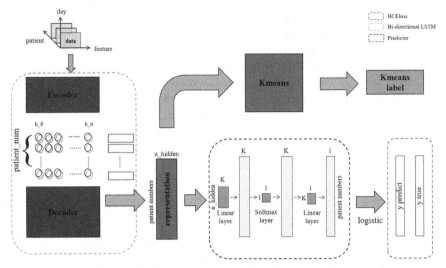

Fig. 3. Algorithm workflow showing how the BiLSTM-AE generated specific representations from the input data in the first step. The second step for clustering and the third step for mortality probability prediction were also performed.

2.4 Statistical Analysis

The distinction among different subphenotypes was explored by statistical analysis after cluster identification. The patient proportion and mortality of different subphenotypes were calculated. For each patient, all measurements' mean values within the first 24 h of presentation were utilized for discussion. In addition, related complication results were utilized to analyze differences between the subphenotypes. The Kruskal-Wallis test was used for continuous variables. Statistical quartile calculations for all values were performed. P < 0.05 was considered statistically significant.

3 Results

3.1 Parameter Selection

To determine the value of k for clustering, which is closely relevant to subphenotypes. The results with different k values, from k = 3 to k = 5, are shown in Fig. 4. The hidden dimensions also needed to be explored. Thus, a two-dimensional parameter space was created including the k value and the number of hidden layers from 3 to 14. The highest silhouette coefficient score was k = 3, with five hidden layers. As a result, k = 3 and five hidden layers were selected to identify sepsis subphenotypes.

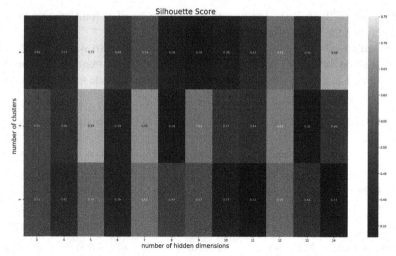

Fig. 4. The results displayed with a heat map. We calculated silhouette coefficient scores of various clustering results under k and hidden layers.

3.2 Subphenotype Characteristics

Of a total of 9,548 events from 1,426 patients during the study period, only 971 patients with 4,905 records met the clustering criteria after data processing and were therefore included in the study. The silhouette coefficient score of $k = 3$ was the highest, as shown in Fig. 4, resulting in three sepsis subphenotypes. There were 748 patients (77.0%) with an overall in-hospital mortality rate of 2.9% in subphenotype 1, 120 (12.4%) with 10.0% mortality rate in subphenotype 2, and 103 (10.6%) with 78.6% mortality rate in subphenotype 3 (Table 1).

The cluster results are shown in Fig. 5. Subphenotype 1 with a 2.94% mortality, subphenotype 2 with a 10.0% mortality, and subphenotype 3 with a 78.64% mortality. Such result demonstrated that there was significant difference among subphenotypes and representations obtained by BiLSTM-AE were associated with mortality.

3.3 Mortality

The area under the receiver operating characteristic curve (AUROC) and the area under precision recall curve (AUPRC) were used to evaluate the predictive performance of our predictor. The AUROC in this study was 0.89, and the AUPRC was 0.65.

3.4 Comparison of Demographic and Physiological Characteristics Between the Subphenotypes

The demographics and physiological characteristics of the three subphenotypes in the study cohort are shown in Table 1. Subphenotype 1 was the youngest, with the mean age of 64.1 years, compared with 67.9 years (subphenotype 2) and 66.2 years (Subphenotype 3). The proportion of men was the highest in subphenotype 3 (subphenotype 1: 52.4%

vs. subphenotype 2: 46.7%). However, there were no significant differences in age and gender between the subphenotypes (P = 0.477).

The median values of the laboratory measurements are also shown in Table 1. We found that some laboratory biomarkers showed a consistent trend, which means that subphenotype 1 had lower values in these features. These include total bilirubin (0.8 vs.

Table 1. Demographic and physiological characteristics between the subphenotypes.

Patient characteristics	Subphenotype 1, N = 748 (77.0%)	Subphenotype 2, n = 120 (12.4%)	Subphenotype 3, n = 103 (10.6%)	P-value
Demographics				
mean age, years	64.1	67.9	66.2	0.031
Men, n (%)	392 (52.4%)	56 (46.7%)	55 (53.4%)	0.477
mortality, n (%)	22 (2.9%)	12 (10.0%)	81 (78.6%)	**<0.001**
Laboratory values, mean (IQR)				
AST (SGOT), units/L	61.0 (20.0–49.0)	75.5 (24.0–71.5)	298.6 (33.0–319.5)	**<0.001**
ALT (SGPT), units/L	49.8 (13.0–34.0)	59.3 (15.0–51.0)	200.2 (28.0–371.0)	**<0.001**
Total bilirubin, mg/dl	0.8 (0.3–0.8)	1.4 (0.4–1.6)	2.8 (0.4–3.7)	**<0.001**
Albumin, g/dl	3.0 (2.7–3.6)	2.6 (2.3–2.8)	2.5 (1.8–3.3)	**<0.001**
BUN, mg/dL	29.2 (15.0–39.0)	40.8 (21.0–50.0)	47.3 (40.0–58.7)	**<0.001**
RDW, %	15.4 (13.7–16.0)	16.8 (14.6–18.1)	17.8 (15.2–18.0)	**<0.001**
Total protein, g/dL	6.1 (5.5–6.8)	5.5 (5.1–6.1)	5.5 (4.5–6.6)	**<0.001**
Glucose, mg/dL	141.1 (111.0–179.0)	150.7 (105.0–182.0)	151.5 (136.3–257.0)	**<0.001**
Hgb, g/dL	10.5 (9.3–12.6)	9.9 (8.6–10.9)	9.7 (8.2–10.2)	**<0.001**
Calcium, mg/dL	8.1 (7.8–8.5)	7.9 (7.2–8.4)	8.1 (6.8–8.1)	0.002
Bedside glucose, mg/dL	146.8 (109.7–167.3)	147.8 (106.2–153.3)	159.5 (124.0–234.7)	0.003
Hct, %	32.2 (28.2–37.6)	30.7 (26.8–33.7)	30.0 (23.9–30.9)	0.004
Creatinine, mg/dl	1.8 (0.9–1.8)	2.3 (1.4–2.6)	2.6 (1.8–3.9)	0.004
Potassium, mmol/L	4.0 (3.7–4.4)	4.2 (3.9–4.8)	4.3 (3.9–5.2)	0.004
RBC, M/µL	3.6 (3.1–4.2)	3.4 (2.9–3.5)	3.3 (2.6–3.7)	0.005
WBC x 1000, K/µL	12.5 (8.9–15.9)	15.7 (11.1–16.6)	15.6 (9.7–22.1)	0.012
Bicarbonate, mmol/L	23.2 (20.0–25.5)	21.1 (17.0–23.5)	21.5 (16.3–26.0)	0.015
Lymphs, %	12.1 (5.9–12.5)	8.4 (3.0–8.6)	10.9 (6.7–11.0)	0.018
Polys, %	75.7 (76.0–87.0)	79.4 (79.0–89.0)	77.6 (67.7–84.2)	0.030

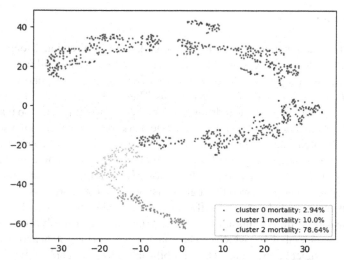

Fig. 5. The clustering results. Subphenotype 1 is in blue, subphenotype 2 is in orange, and subphenotype 3 is in green.

1.4 vs. 2.8, mg/dL; P < 0.001), BUN (29.2 vs. 40.8 vs. 47.3, mg/dL; P < 0.001), RDW (15.4 vs. 16.8 vs. 17.8, %; P < 0.01), AST (SGOT) (61.0 vs. 75.5 vs. 298.6, units/L; P < 0.001), ALT (SGPT) (49.8 vs. 59.3 vs. 200.2, units/L; P < 0.001), and glucose (141.1 vs. 150.7 vs. 151.5, mg/dL; P < 0.001). Hgb (10.5 vs. 9.9 vs. 9.7, g/dL), albumin (3.0 vs. 2.6 vs. 2.5, g/dL), and total protein (6.1 vs. 5.5 vs. 5.5, g/dL) were highest in subphenotype 1, which demonstrated significant difference (P < 0.001). Other biomarkers are also displayed in Table 1. All biomarkers in Table 1 were utilized to create violin plots (Fig. 6).

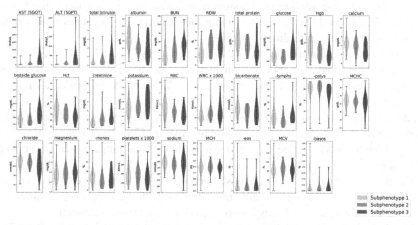

Fig. 6. Violin plots for 29 features. Subphenotype 1 is shown in red, subphenotype 2 is in green, and subphenotype 3 is in purple. Definition of abbreviations: AST, aspartate transaminase; ALT, alanine transaminase; BUN, urea nitrogen; RDW, red blood cell distribution width; Hgb, hemoglobin; Hct, hematocrit; RBC, red blood cell; WBC × 1000, white blood cells; lymphs, lymphocytes; polys, polymorphonuclear neutrophils. (Color figure online)

4 Discussion

In this study, a new patient subtyping framework with bi-directional long short-term memory Auto-Encoder (BiLSTM-AE) together with k-means algorithm was proposed to identify subphenotypes in patients with sepsis. Three distinct subphenotypes were discovered with distinct organ dysfunction patterns. These subphenotypes differ remarkably in demographic and physiological differences as well as mortality. The top features with greatest difference among subphnotypes include markers of liver function, such as albumin and total protein, and erythrocyte markers. Our approach showed robust associations between the three subphenotypes of sepsis and poor hospital outcomes in a large ICU cohort. We found that subphenotype 1 had a low risk, with the mortality rate of 2.9%, whereas subphenotype 3 showed the highest risk with 78.6% mortality.

The top features with greatest difference among subphnotypes include Bilirubin, BUN and aspartate transaminase and alanine transaminase. Bilirubin is a breakdown product of heme metabolism, which can be transformed into the potent antioxidant under specific physiological conditions [1]. Total bilirubin level of subphenotype 3 with the mean age of 66.2 years was the highest. It has been shown [17] that there is a significant correlation between ethnicity and total bilirubin levels with total mortality. Lower as well as higher levels of total bilirubin are remarkably associated with a higher mortality risk. Furthermore, bilirubin levels generally increase with age. However, other studies did not report the effects of elevated bilirubin on survival [18]. This may be because of distinct baseline for individuals of different races and ages, which could also explain why it was difficult to distinguish sepsis subphenotypes based on bilirubin as a biomarker.

A multicenter observation study has shown that elevated BUN is linked to increased mortality in a certain range of creatinine, and it could presumably be a marker reflecting mortality in critically ill patients [19]. Some risk prediction models, such as those for myocardial infarction [20], include BUN. BUN was also utilized for predicting short-term mortality in patients with severe acute kidney injury who required dialysis [21]. In our study, this marker in subphenotype 3 was significantly the highest, which means that BUN could potentially determine subphenotypes of sepsis as well as predict subphenotype-specific mortality.

Furthermore, there were several fold differences in AST and ALT between the subphenotypes. These two markers were considered predictors of clinical outcomes such as mortality in previous work [22]. Hence, AST and ALT were crucial in identifying sepsis subphenotypes.

Albumin and total protein are closely related to liver function, and albumin may be a highly sensitive indicator of clinical disease severity [23]. Both indicators were the lowest in subphenotype 3 and were not within the normal range, revealing abnormal liver function.

The three subphenotypes generally showed hemoglobin, hematocrit, and red blood cells below the normal range, where subphenotype 3 showed the lowest values. This suggests that subphenotype 3 may be associated with more severe anemia.

The limitations of this study stem from partial population inclusion in eICU. These conclusions are only based on the conclusions of preliminary experiments, and more populations are still needed to verify the conclusions. In addition, an externally validated argument is necessary.

In conclusion, three subphenotypes in patients with sepsis were discovered using the newly proposed framework. This framework is not only able to identify subphenotypes, but also predicts the mortality. The results in this study suggest that physiological differences between these three subphenotypes probably lead to various treatment, which may drive personalization of sepsis management.

Funding. This research was supported by the Key Discipline Fund of Shenzhen Hospital of Southern Medical University (No. 2021-2023ICU).

Ethics. Publicly available datasets with preexisting ethics approvals from the original studies were used in this work. All researchers in this project hold a CITI certificate.

References

1. Hotchkiss, R.S., Karl, I.E.: The pathophysiology and treatment of sepsis. N. Engl. J. Med. **348**, 138–150 (2003)
2. Gullo, A., Bianco, N., Berlot, G.: Management of severe sepsis and septic shock: challenges and recommendations. Crit. Care Clin. **22**, 489–501, ix (2006)
3. Angus, D.C., Linde-Zwirble, W.T., Lidicker, J., Clermont, G., Carcillo, J., Pinsky, M.R.: Epidemiology of severe sepsis in the United States: analysis of incidence, outcome, and associated costs of care. Crit. Care Med. **29**, 1303–1310 (2001)
4. Nemati, S., Holder, A., Razmi, F., Stanley, M.D., Clifford, G.D., Buchman, T.G.: An Interpretable machine learning model for accurate prediction of sepsis in the ICU. Crit. Care Med. **46**, 547–553 (2018)
5. Kam, H.J., Kim, H.Y.: Learning representations for the early detection of sepsis with deep neural networks. Comput. Biol. Med. **89**, 248–255 (2017)
6. Bhavani, S.V., Carey, K.A., Gilbert, E.R., Afshar, M., Verhoef, P.A., Churpek, M.M.: Identifying novel sepsis subphenotypes using temperature trajectories. Am. J. Respir. Crit. Care Med. **200**, 327–335 (2019)
7. Yin, C.C., Liu, R.Q., Zhang, D.D., Zhang, P.: Identifying sepsis subphenotypes via time-aware multi-modal auto-encoder. In: KDD 2020: Proceedings of the 26th ACM SIGKDD International Conference on Knowledge Discovery & Data Mining, pp. 862–872 (2020)
8. Sinha, P., Delucchi, K.L., Thompson, B.T., McAuley, D.F., Matthay, M.A., Calfee, C.S.: Latent class analysis of ARDS subphenotypes: a secondary analysis of the statins for acutely injured lungs from sepsis (SAILS) study. Intensive Care Med. **44**(11), 1859–1869 (2018). https://doi.org/10.1007/s00134-018-5378-3
9. Maddali, M.V., et al.: Validation and utility of ARDS subphenotypes identified by machine-learning models using clinical data: an observational, multicohort, retrospective analysis. Lancet Respir. Med. **10**, 367–377 (2022)
10. Pollard, T.J., Johnson, A.E.W., Raffa, J.D., Celi, L.A., Mark, R.G., Badawi, O.: The eICU Collaborative research database, a freely available multi-center database for critical care research. Sci. Data **5**, 180178 (2018)
11. Huang, H.F., Liu, Y., Wu, M., Gao, Y., Yu, X.X.: Development and validation of a risk stratification model for predicting the mortality of acute kidney injury in critical care patients. Ann. Transl. Med. **9** (2021)
12. Singer, M., et al.: The third international consensus definitions for sepsis and septic shock (sepsis-3). JAMA **315**, 801–810 (2016)
13. Siami-Namini, S., Tavakoli, N., Namin, A.S.: The performance of LSTM and BiLSTM in forecasting time series. In: IEEE International Conference on Big Data, pp. 3285–3292 (2019)

14. Hochreiter, S., Schmidhuber, J.: Long short-term memory. Neural Comput. **9**, 1735–1780 (1997)

15. Hartigan, J.A., Wong, M.A.: Algorithm AS 136: a k-means clustering algorithm. J. R. Stat. Soc. Ser. c (Appl. Stat.) **28**, 100–108 (1979)

16. van der Maaten, L., Hinton, G.: Visualizing data using t-SNE. J. Mach. Learn. Res. **9**, 2579–2605 (2008)

17. Ong, K.L., Allison, M.A., Cheung, B.M.Y., Wu, B., Barter, P.J., Rye, K.A.: The relationship between total bilirubin levels and total mortality in older adults: the United States National Health and Nutrition Examination Survey (NHANES). PLoS ONE **9**, 1999–2004 (2014)

18. Boland, B.S., Dong, M.H., Bettencourt, R., Barrett-Connor, E., Loomba, R.: Association of serum bilirubin with aging and mortality. J. Clin. Exp. Hepatol. **4**, 1–7 (2014)

19. Beier, K., et al.: Elevation of blood urea nitrogen is predictive of long-term mortality in critically ill patients independent of "normal" creatinine. Crit. Care Med. **39**, 305–313 (2011)

20. Luria, M.H., Knoke, J.D., Margolis, R.M., Hendricks, F.H., Kuplic, J.B.: Acute myocardial infarction: prognosis after recovery. Ann. Intern. Med. **85**, 561–565 (1976)

21. Liu, K.D., et al.: Timing of initiation of dialysis in critically ill patients with acute kidney injury. Clin. J. Am. Soc. Nephrol. **1**, 915–919 (2006)

22. Wang, Y., Shi, L., Wang, Y., Yang, H.: An updated meta-analysis of AST and ALT levels and the mortality of COVID-19 patients. Am. J. Emerg. Med. **40**, 208–209 (2021)

23. Goldwasser, P., Feldman, J.: Association of serum albumin and mortality risk. J. Clin. Epidemiol. **50**, 693–703 (1997)

Machine Learning for Multimodal Electronic Health Records-Based Research: Challenges and Perspectives

Ziyi Liu[1,2], Jiaqi Zhang[1], Yongshuai Hou[1], Xinran Zhang[1,3], Ge Li[4],
and Yang Xiang[1(✉)]

[1] Department of Network Intelligence, Peng Cheng Laboratory, Shenzhen, China
ziyiliu@andrew.cmu.edu, {zhangjq02,houysh,xiangy}@pcl.ac.cn,
xinran.zhang@mail.utoronto.ca
[2] School of Computer Science, Carnegie Mellon University, Pittsburgh, USA
[3] Mathematical and Computational Sciences, University of Toronto Mississauga, Mississauga,
Canada
[4] School of Electronic and Computer Engineering, Peking University, Shenzhen, China
lige@pcl.ac.cn

Abstract. Electronic Health Records (EHRs) contain rich information of patient health status, which usually include both structured and unstructured data. There have been many studies focusing on distilling valuable information from structured data, such as disease codes, laboratory test results, and treatments. However, relying on structured data only might be insufficient in reflecting patients' comprehensive information and such data may occasionally contain erroneous records. With the recent advances of machine learning (ML) and deep learning (DL) techniques, an increasing number of studies seek to obtain more accurate results by incorporating unstructured free-text data as well. This paper reviews studies that use multimodal data, i.e. a combination of structured and unstructured data, from EHRs as input for conventional ML or DL models to address the targeted tasks. We searched in the Institute of Electrical and Electronics Engineers (IEEE) Digital Library, PubMed, and Association for Computing Machinery (ACM) Digital Library for articles related to ML and DL-based multimodal EHR studies. With the final 94 included studies, we focus on how EHR data from different modalities were combined and interacted using conventional ML and DL techniques, the influence of the relationship between multimodal data on their fusion strategy, and how these algorithms were applied in EHR-related tasks. Further, we investigate the advantages and limitations of these fusion methods and indicate future directions for ML-based multimodal EHR research.

Keywords: Machine learning · Deep learning · Electronic health records · Multimodal

---

Z. Liu and J. Zhang—Equal contribution.

B. Tang et al. (Eds.): CHIP 2022, CCIS 1772, pp. 135–155, 2023.
https://doi.org/10.1007/978-981-19-9865-2_10

1 Introduction

Electronic Health Records (EHRs) offer an efficient way to maintain patient information and are becoming more and more widely used by healthcare providers around the world [1]. Both structured and unstructured free-text data could be stored in EHRs in an organized way. Structured data can include numerical data such as lab test results, coded data such as procedure codes and diagnosis codes, categorical data such as medication lists and vital signs, and demographic information. Unstructured data such as clinical notes and discharge summaries can record more expressive and detailed descriptions of the patient' s pain level, differences from the last visit, unique characteristics of their case, and anything that the physician thinks might be helpful for diagnosis and treatment, and supplement the nuances not seen in structured data [2]. For example, Fox et al. validated a sample of hip fracture medical records and showed that coded records only have 66.7% sensitivity and 78.9% specificity for representing complications compared to postoperative notes [3]. By means of EHRs, physicians are able to keep track of patients' health status and visit history to facilitate diagnosis. Meanwhile, informaticians could develop algorithms to extract patterns from the vast amount of medical data of EHRs and provide insightful suggestions to physicians' decision-making [4, 5].

Machine learning (ML) have been used in a broad range of predictive tasks in healthcare, e.g. drug-drug interaction recognition, [6] disease progress prediction [7] and tumor detection [8]. In the past decades, traditional ML methods for EHR mining focused primarily on using structured data, which can usually be easily processed and analyzed using computer programs, and have demonstrated the effectiveness of corresponding predictive variables [4, 9]. However, such structured data may suffer from missing- or erroneous-value problems, and thus cannot always guarantee consistent and accurate prediction results when used alone, as pointed out by [10, 11]. Unstructured free-text data are harder to understand by programs, but are less prone to such errors, and it has been shown that textual features extracted by Natural Language Processing (NLP) pipelines can lead to positive results and serve as compensation to structured features [12]. With the development of more advanced ML and deep learning (DL) techniques, studies started to merge the two modalities, which are complementary in nature, to fully exploit the predictive potential of EHRs. Modality fusion strategies play a significant role in these studies.

There have been many reviews summarizing studies with EHR data as shown in Table 1. However, most reviews either do not discuss the fusion strategies of modalities [13–15] or focus on conventional ML methods only. [12, 16–18] discusses fusion strategies in DL, but is of structured data and imaging data. In addition, some reviews are limited to one type of disease [12] or one type of task [12, 15, 16]. In our paper, we focus exclusively on studies that use conventional ML and DL techniques with multimodal EHR data, and place our emphasis on the strategies for combining textual data from different modalities. This definition of multimodality within this paper refers to structured data and unstructured free-texts in EHRs, which is converging with heterogeneity, but different from the traditional definition that often also includes audio, image, and videos as data sources. We don' t place restrictions on certain types of diseases or tasks.

In the following sections, we review the cohort that supports multimodal analysis, tasks that involve multimodal analysis, and ML models and fusion strategies used in these studies. We also introduce a new taxonomy, i.e. interaction strategies, that is targeted to aligning the simple-form structured data to different processing granularities of unstructured data beyond fusion strategies, aiming at categorizing the fusion styles from the semantic level. We thus provide a comprehensive analysis of recent progress in multimodal EHR analysis. In addition, we summarize the limitations of these methodologies and present potential future directions in this field. We expect that through this review, researchers can have a thorough view of the advancement of ML techniques in combing multimodal EHRs and a better understanding of how ML and DL models could be designed to align textual data from different modalities.

Table 1. Existing reviews with similar studied aspects.

	Modalities of included studies	ML/DL	Main focus and whether modality fusion discussed	Task
Shickel 2018 [13]	Primarily structured + a few with both structured and unstructured	DL	DL techniques and their application to different HER - based clinical tasks. Presents modality fusion as future direction	All clinical tasks regardless of application domain
Xiao 2018 [14]	Primarily structured + a few with both structured and unstructured	DL	Identifying analytical tasks and introduces commonly used models for each task. Presents modality fusion as future direction	All clinical tasks regardless of application domain
Huang 2020 [18]	Imaging + structured data	DL	Fusion strategies of the modalities and implementation guidelines of multimodal models	All clinical tasks regardless of application domain
Si 2021 [15]	Multimodal	DL	Resources, methods, applications and potential of EHR representation learning Presents modality fusion as future direction	All representation learning studies regardless of application domain
Sheikhalishahi 2019 [17]	Clinical notes	ML + three DL articles	Application of NLP to clinical notes in 10 different chronic diseases groups Does not discuss modality fusion	Chronic diseases
Zeng 2019 [16]	Primarily structured + a few with both structured and unstructured	Rule-based, ML, DL	Application and state-of-the-art of NLP methods for computational phenotyping. Presents modality fusion as future direction	Six tasks of computational phenotyping regardless of application domain

(continued)

Table 1. (*continued*)

	Modalities of included studies	ML/DL	Main focus and whether modality fusion discussed	Task
Ford 2016 [12]	Primarily multimodal + a few with unstructured only	Rule-based, ML	Information extraction methods from unstructured data and improvement over structured data only Does not focus on modality fusion	Case-detection for named clinical conditions

2 Search Methods

The focus of this methodological review is on the application of conventional ML and DL techniques to multimodal EHR-based tasks, in which multimodal is defined as including both structured and unstructured free-text data. To obtain the set of related articles, we followed a PRISMA-like style and first searched in Institute of Electrical and Electronics Engineers (IEEE) Digital Library, PubMed, and Association for Computing Machinery (ACM) Digital Library with the key concepts multimodal, EHR, machine learning, and deep learning to form the query keywords. We used various forms of each keyword, and included different ML and DL algorithms, shown in Table 2. The search resulted in 677 studies. Our inclusion criteria are that the research study must be using both structured and unstructured free-text EHR data in the proposed model, and that the model must use conventional ML or DL techniques. Based on these criteria, we screened 222 articles according to the title and abstract at the first step, and after full-text review, 82 articles were left. We then snowballed on other relevant review articles and included studies. Our final pool has 94 studies.

Table 2. Detailed searching query.

Part name	Query
Multimodal data	(multimodal OR multi-modal OR multi-modality OR "multi modal" OR heterogeneous OR unstructured OR notes OR texts OR sequential OR "time series") NOT (image OR imaging)
EHR	(ehr OR "electronic health records" OR emr OR "electronic medical records")
Deep learning	("deep learning" OR "deep representation" OR "neural network" OR embedding OR convolutional OR recurrent OR autoencoder OR "long short-term memory" OR transformer OR "restricted boltzmann" OR "generative adversarial" OR "multilayer perceptron")
Machine learning	("machine learning" OR "svm" OR "support vector machine" OR "logistic regression" OR "decision tree" OR "lr" OR "dt")

During the full-text review, we analyzed the studies from three perspectives: data, task, and model. For data, we focus on two parts, the first is the dataset used by the studies, including size, language, availability and data types used (categorical, numerical, free-text, etc.), and the second part is the relationship between the different modal data in the data used, and how this relationship affects their fusion strategy. For task, we looked at where and how the proposed model is applied, and summarized the task type. Finally, for model, we focused on the fusion strategy of modalities, and recorded the algorithm type of each model.

3   Results

3.1   Cohorts

The population size in each study varies greatly from hundreds to millions (of patients). For example, [19] used a dataset with only 300 patients to train a complex disease identification model, while [20] used a dataset of 6 million patients for atopic dermatitis identification. The dataset size used in most studies (83.0%, 78/94) is over 1,000. Cohorts from large datasets were mostly generated automatically according to certain criteria (i.e. phenotyping) related to the research aims, [21] while the cohorts from most small datasets were often manually chosen and annotated, which could have higher accuracy and be more targeted towards their tasks. [22] Moreover, most (66.7%, 52/78) large datasets (e.g. >1000) are in English with data from the US and UK, and datasets in other languages such as Chinese, [23] Dutch, [24] Swedish, [25, 26] and Japanese [26] tend to be smaller.

The multimodal EHR datasets generally contain clinical text (e.g. clinical notes), codes (e.g. ICD codes), categorical data (e.g. medication list), and numerical data (e.g. laboratory measurements). More than half of the studied datasets (52.1%, 49/94) include multi-visit sequential information, although some proposed models did not specifically model such information. [20, 22, 27] Most studies used private datasets or did not mention the availability (81.9%, 77/94), while others used publicly available datasets [28–30] or shared their datasets. [21, 31] The most popular (14.9%, 14/94) public dataset is the Medical Information Mart for Intensive Care III (MIMIC-III), which comprises de-identified health-related data associated with 53,423 distinct hospital admissions for adult patients. [32] Other public datasets such as Vanderbilt University Medical Center EHR, [33] Mount Sinai Data Warehouse [34] and I2B2 [35] were also used more than once in the included studies and can be used to conduct further multimodal EHR research.

3.2   Relationships Between Modalities

Coded data (e.g. procedure codes and diagnosis codes) are widely used in EHRs and contain rich information about patients, such as symptoms and medical diagnoses. Clinical text and diagnosis codes are the most frequently used EHR data types in the analyzed papers. The relationships between clinical text and coded data can be broadly classified into three categories, (a) textual data contain or describe coded data, (b) coded data summarize textual data, e.g. ICD codes and corresponding symptom diagnosis description, and (c) coded data are independent of textual data, each describing different information about patients. These three different categories elaborate the containment relationships between unstructured text information and medical coded data in EHR. These two types of data have different content and scope of information expressed from different perspectives, which can provide clues to the design of different fusion strategies in ML-based methods.

In the first category where textual data contain diagnosis codes, coded data usually exist as phrases in unstructured textual data. Because such EHR data directly contains the patient's diagnostic information, coded data often becomes an important field for expressing rich semantic information in unstructured text data. In the second category, structured coded data are stored as separate structured data in EHR, which is one of the most common cases in EHR tasks. In this category, coded data are often treated as an essential information field for individual embedding operations and have important references to the corresponding textual information both in the pre-sample screening phase and in the subsequent conventional ML or DL process. The combination of ICD code information with textual data containing corresponding symptom descriptions was used in the study by DeLisle et al. This fusion was shown to help improve detection sensitivity [89]. Typically, the relationship between diagnosis codes and textual data fall into the first two cases, but other coded data may fall more into the third category. The third category is where coded data are independent of textual information. In this case, the two types of data can be considered as complementary to each other without intersection and therefore should be encoded as equally important and the information contained in the two kinds of data should be integrated in the subsequent learning process. For example, Hu et al. used feature-level join operations for both types of data in this context to accomplish the integration of the two kinds of information [29].

3.3 Tasks

Traditional ML-based tasks related to EHRs can be roughly divided into clinical information regularization and clinical decision-making. Usually, unstructured information, such as case reports and nursing notes, is used as the main data source in the former type of task. The information is extracted through NLP processes and transformed into a structured format that is easier to store and analyze [36]. In comparison, for the latter task, structured information such as ICD codes and patient demographics data is more often used [37, 38]. Informaticians have also been exploring the fusion of the two types of information. For example, Payrovnaziri and Barrett extended their prior work by adding unstructured text features into previously used structured data to predict one-year mortality risk of patients with acute myocardial infarction [39]. Experiments demonstrate that the performance of the algorithmic model that combines both structured and unstructured information is superior to the results obtained when only one of them is used [40].

According to our review, multimodal data that combine structured and unstructured information are currently mainly used in the clinical decision-making task (47.9%, 45/94), e.g. the prediction of a disease [41–44]. The second popular direction is identifying cohorts using phenotyping algorithms, which also accounts for a big proportion (30.9%, 29/94). Another direction, which is more related to the clinical information regularization task is patient representation learning (6.4%, 6/94), where researchers attempt to model multimodal EHR data in a shared semantic space for general clinical tasks [28]. The effectiveness of these learned representations is verified on baseline tasks such as the prediction of hospital length of stay and the rate of readmission, and shows that representations learned from multimodal data have a more comprehensive generalization ability in solving real-world problems [7]. These studies may provide further directions on applicable scenarios of multimodal data for EHR researchers, and the improved performances on a wide range of tasks have demonstrated the properness and explorable space of this direction.

3.4 Machine Learning Methods

In total, there are 65 (69.1%) papers primarily using conventional ML and 29 (30.9%) papers primarily using DL. As discussed above, most tasks with multimodal EHR deal with classification (clinical decision-making and phenotyping) or patient representation problems. For classification tasks such as disease prediction and risk assessment, relevant studies used mainly (70.7%, 53/75) conventional ML models, such as Logistic Regression (LR), [20, 46, 47] Random Forest (RF), [21, 46, 48] Support Vector Machines (SVMs), [29, 49, 50] and Naive Bayes (NB) [27, 49, 50]. For instance, Chen et al. took the UMLS concepts extracted from clinical notes and billing codes as input and incorporated active learning to SVM-based phenotyping algorithms [51]. Slightly different from traditional approaches, Zhao and Weng designed a weighted Bayesian Network Inference (BNI) model where they combined structured EHR data with a prior probability calculated from free-text PubMed abstracts of the expert selected variables for pancreatic cancer prediction [52].

Despite the popularity of conventional ML for classification tasks, DL models were greatly explored over the recent years, and are being applied to both classification tasks and representation learning tasks. (Fig. 1 illustrates the percentage of DL over years) [53–55] CNN has been shown to be good at extracting locality-invariant features, which can be useful for identifying key concepts in clinical notes [56]. On the other hand, RNN, and especially its variant Long Short-Term Memory Networks (LSTM), [57] is well known for discovering sequential dependencies, which is often used to model clinical notes (text as sequence) and temporal information in EHR [28]. More recently, Transformer-based pre-trained models are also adapted to the medical domain. Huang et al. developed ClinicalBERT, which pre-trained the BERT model on clinical notes in MIMIC-III [58]. This model has also been used by many multimodal EHR studies to build embeddings for free-text data [43, 45, 59]. Among the included studies, BERT [43] and word embeddings [71] are the most commonly used techniques to compute the representation [34]. Other approaches that applied recent DL techniques also exist. Lee et al. built a harmonized representation space for patients, medical concepts and medical events by modeling the time-variant patient' s nodes with LSTM, and time-invariant concept and event nodes with Graph Convolutional Networks (GCN), which fused multimodal inputs [60]. After obtaining these representations, they can be used as input to both conventional ML and DL models for downstream tasks.

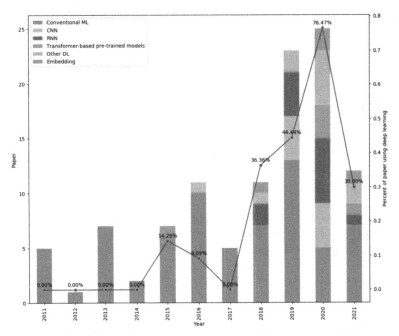

Fig. 1. Different methods used in the research papers, and the percentage of DL over years.

To compare, most conventional ML methods take each feature, either from structured or unstructured EHRs, independently owing to their shallow structures. For example, it is hard for RF and SVM to capture the sequential dependencies conveyed in unstructured data, and thus some deeper semantic information might be missed during modeling. On the other hand, DL models have a stronger capacity to model different levels of dependencies between feature dimensions so that complex interactions between modalities might be built. Specifically, DL models are superior in modeling free-text, e.g. using semantic structures and embeddings, which is more conformable with the nature of free-text.

3.5 Fusion Strategies

The remarkable characteristic of multimodal EHR research is that useful information can be conveyed by both structured and unstructured data, and thus features extracted from the two modalities should be fused effectively. As a reference, there exists a generally accepted taxonomy by previous studies which categorizes multimodal data fusion in ML into three types: early fusion, joint fusion, and late fusion, as shown in Fig. 2 [18]. We firstly tried to align each study to this taxonomy, shown in Table 3.

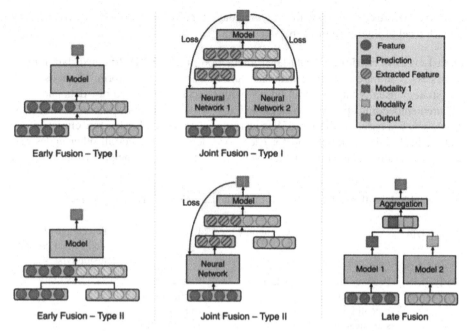

Fig. 2. Early/joint/late fusion by Huang et al. 2020 [18].

3.6 Interaction Strategies

Unlike imaging and speech data which usually need to be preprocessed separately and transformed into feature vectors before fusion, free-text data are more flexible in the sense that its fusion with structured data can start at a much earlier stage and be in a more direct way because of the similarity in modality. Each word in free-text is semantically meaningful by itself, whereas extracting such segments from an image or a speech signal sequence often requires additional handling. Different levels of text processing could lead to features capturing different granularities of semantics. For example, raw free-text data could be used directly to compute word embeddings that can reflect relationships between words, and concepts and topics could be extracted from free-text to represent its meaning at the sentence/document level.

Therefore, as free-text data has higher granularities, the three fusion strategies alone might be insufficient to fully represent the various levels of interactions between multi modalities. For example, using raw words, word embeddings or named entities with codes as the combined input to a neural network model can all be aligned to early fusion, but they represent quite distinct combination scenarios where different complementary and interdependent information could be carried and different model structures could be applied. We design a novel and finer-grained taxonomy, interaction strategies, to better represent how multimodal data are fused and help us understand better how different models deal with multimodal data according to their operational mechanism from the semantic level. We define five categories based on the degree to which free-text data is processed before combining with structured data (Fig. 3). We also discuss pros and cons of each level of interaction in Table 4.

Data-Level Interaction. In data-level interaction (4.2%, 3/94), free-text data remain unprocessed and are combined with structured data in their raw form. Methods using this strategy usually take as input both structured and unstructured raw data and learn a shared embedding space by word embedding models. Bai et al. proposed JointSkip-gram, which is based on the Word2Vec learning schema [71]. It takes raw clinical notes and medical codes as input, and for each code, learns to predict all other codes and words in the same visit, while for each word, learns to predict its neighboring words and

Table 3. Different fusion types for multimodal EHR data that can be aligned to.

Fusion type	Definition	Commonly used by	Examples	Percentage of studies that use the fusion type
Early fusion	Features are extracted from modalities by statistical methods, existing NLP tools, word embedding models, or other DL models, and combined prior to passing to the model	ML, DL	Statistical methods [26, 48, 61] Existing NLP tools [21, 46, 62] Word embedding models [39, 63, 64] Other DL models [22, 59, 65]	88.3%, 83/94
Joint fusion	Combines the modalities at intermediary layers of the neural network, and losses can be propagated back to the feature extraction phase to dynamically update the feature weights	DL	[31, 66–68]	7.4%, 7/94
Late fusion	Separate models are used for each modality, and the final decision leverages the decision of each individual model by some ensemble strategies	ML	[48, 63, 69, 70]	6.3%, 4/94

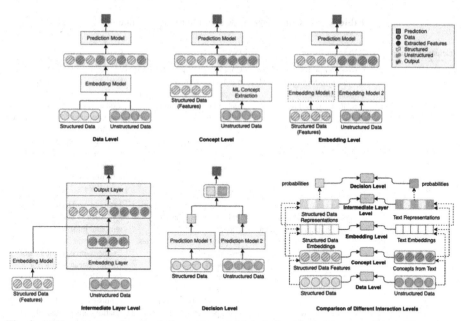

Fig. 3. Different interaction levels for multimodal data fusion. Dotted boxes and dotted lines mean optional. We also demonstrate the comparison of different interaction levels in the last sub-figure. The legend is similar to that in Fig. 2.

all codes. The resulting representation is able to capture not only similarities within the same modality, but also cross different modalities through shared weights.

Concept-Level Interaction. Concept-level interaction (74.5%, 70/94) refers to extracting features firstly by statistics or established packages from each modality, and combining them using simple ways such as concatenation. As the free-text features can be either raw data or clinical concepts, e.g. named entities, we call this interaction concept-level. This is a typical type of early fusion, and appears most often in conventional ML studies, before the advance of DL. Feature values of structured data are often represented as the frequencies of events, while for free-text data, they are extracted using Term Frequency-Inverse Document Frequency (TF-IDF), bag of words, topic modeling methods such as Latent Dirichlet Allocation (LDA), [72] or established NLP pipelines such as clinical Text Analysis and Knowledge Extraction System (cTAKES), [73] MetaMap, [74] KnowledgeMap, [75] and Health Information Text Extraction (HITEx). [62, 76] is a typical example of concept-level interaction with ML, where features such as disease concepts, lab results, and medications were extracted from both codified structured data and clinical notes using HITEx. Then the frequencies of events were passed to penalized logistic regression to predict rheumatoid arthritis.

Table 4. Pros and cons of the five interaction strategies.

Interaction strategy	Example usage	Pros	Cons
Data-level	Consider both words and clinical codes as tokens. Mix them and explore their relations according to co-occurrence	Could lead to the discovery of mutual and representative features which are present in more than one modality	1) Data from the two modalities are considered as coming from only one modality, e.g. consider a code as a word, thus discrimination is ignored 2) Resulting representation is more likely to capture shared rather than complementary information from the modalities
Concept-level	Extract clinical entities as concepts from text and combine them with clinical codes	1) Can be easily implemented and is computationally efficient 2) Extracted textual features provide a clean and concise representation of the unstructured data, and thus increases the model's interpretability and is useful when performing feature analysis and ablation study	1) Could lead to information loss, such as contextual and temporal information in free-text data 2) The routine method using simple concatenation is a relatively naive way to combine modalities that cannot exploit full relationships between the modalities
Embedding-level	Embed both words and clinical codes as vectors and serve them as inputs to a neural network	1) Word embeddings and neural networks can greatly preserve information in free-text and well-formed patterns and features in structured data could be discovered than using frequency counts 2) Dependency on external tools is reduced	1) The boundary between modalities is blurred with concatenated single-modal representations, which might cause the model to rely on dominating modality instead of learning the cross-modality interaction 2) Decreased model interpretability
Intermediate Layer-level	Encode texts using a neural network and combine with clinical codes at a non-output layer	1) Retains all advantages of embedding-level interaction and provides better interaction flexibility 2) Easier to learn complementary information from all modalities and dynamically update feature weights accordingly by incorporating the combination step within the model	1) Low quality features from one modality could be harmful and add additional noise to the model 2) It is debatable whether one or two layers could fully capture the complex relationships between the modalities depending on at which layer the interaction happens
Decision-level	Build deterministic models for each modality and average the outputs of both	Performance of each modality can be evaluated separately, which can be useful when the number of modalities is large, or there are multichannel representations, and decisions need to be made regarding which ones to keep	Models in this interaction strategy are not exposed to multimodal data at all, and thus may not be able to effectively use the rich information contained in the multimodal data and capture the latent interactions between

Embedding-Level Interaction. Embedding-level interaction (18.1%, 17/94) shows another way of integrating free-text, in which representations of free-text data are obtained by passing the raw text through a pre-trained word embedding or neural network model. Structured data can be represented similarly as in concept-level interaction or also be passed through a neural network model as embedding-like representations. The embedding vectors from each modality are then concatenated or summed up as the input for the final output model. This type of interaction is used by many DL studies according to our review due to the ability of embeddings to capture more comprehensive information from the raw data. Beeksma et al. embedded unstructured free-text data using Word2Vec, and concatenated with structured codes, laboratory, and medication data for life expectancy prediction using LSTM [64]. Darabi et al. developed two separate modules for code and text representation [59]. The code module is composed of a skip-gram model followed by a Transformer encoder [77] and the text module uses BioBERT followed by a Bi-GRU. Finally, the patient representation is a concatenation of the code and text representations.

Intermediate Layer-Level Interaction. In intermediate layer-level interaction (4.3%, 4/94), the interaction of modalities happens between the embedding and the output layer. Intermediate layer-level interaction is used only by DL studies, but less popular than embedding-level interaction. Liu et al. proposed CNN- and Bi- LSTM-based models for chronic disease prediction, which first represented free-text data using word embedding pre-trained on medical data, and passed to the base model [31]. Structured data were concatenated to the layer before the last fully connected layer. Xu et al. adopted a novel approach with Memory Networks, where they used clinical notes encoded by hierarchical LSTM as the query, and fed structured clinical sequences into the memory [42]. Then the information similar to the query (unstructured data) is extracted from the memory (structured data) and combined with the query to form a representation for acute kidney injury predictions.

Decision-Level Interaction. Decision-level interaction (4.3%, 4/94) is the same as late fusion, in which separate models are built for each modality, and modalities only interact with each other after each output layer. Shin et al. used TF-IDF and topic modeling to represent two types of clinical notes, and built separate logistic regression models for each feature set [69]. The final division is the average of all model outputs. This level of interaction is not commonly used in multimodal EHR studies, especially those with DL.

In addition to these semantic granularity-based interactions, there also are interaction scenarios that are specific to EHRs and from other perspectives. For example, the multimodal data can be fused in either the visit level, i.e. the interaction happens within each visit, or the patient level, i.e. the interaction happens after all the visits are encoded. In these scenarios, either of the above-mentioned interactions on different levels could be leveraged.

4   Limitations

The acquisition of multimodal EHR data is one of the most significant limitations. Since different EHR systems have different standards, not all systems store data as having both "structured" and "unstructured" parts, especially in different countries, where data might be all structured, all semi-structured, or all unstructured. This makes multimodal EHR datasets more scarce than single-modal data. And as mentioned in the cohort section, most current multimodal EHR data are in English, it could introduce distribution biases on population that might lead to algorithmic biases. Finally, unlike structured data, unstructured data is more sensitive to the missing data problem. It is possible to impute a missing blood pressure value, but difficult to impute a missing clinical note.

Another limitation is on the modality interaction techniques and models used. Although the advance of DL propels new techniques such as embedding and intermediate layer level interaction, the "interaction" strategy in these studies is still simple and possibly insufficient to capture complex interactions between different modalities. In addition, base models in these studies are often restricted to traditional ML and simple DL models. This could be due to the fact that processing and extracting useful information from free-text data by traditional informaticians, statisticians or physicians remains a challenge. There have been studies using more complex models such as Graph Convolutional Networks to wrap up data from multimodalities, [60] but the number remains limited, and the exploration is still incipient.

5 Future Directions

5.1 Include More Data Modalities

Although we focus on structured and unstructured text as our multimodal data, other modalities such as images and videos could also be integrated using the aforementioned fusion or interaction techniques [18, 78]. Integrating more data modalities could be helpful if each data modality contains incomplete but complementary information, which is frequently seen in EHRs. For example, patient history, imaging diagnostic report and associated lab test values could naturally be used together with medical imaging for making clinical decisions [78]. However, whether to include data from more sources is also restricted by the data availability and sharing policies in many cases. Furthermore, in some scenarios, prior knowledge, including terminologies, ontologies and knowledge bases, have also been proven useful when performing ML-aided clinical prediction [52, 68]. It can serve as another data modality and the relevant techniques deserve a deeper investigation.

5.2 Enable More Flexible Data Acquisition and Sharing

As mentioned above, the availability of multimodal data is one of the limitations that hinder the development of corresponding research. There are many factors (e.g. gender, ethnicity, political issues, weather, region, environmental humidity) that could influence the research directions or even clinical decisions, it might not be sufficient to rely on the few public datasets to make conclusive clinical claims to the general population. Therefore, it is necessary to encourage more institutions or hospitals to share flexible data to include a more general and broader range of population to facilitate clinical research. In ML, federated learning (FL) [88] has the capability to collect patients' data with the safety of patients' privacy protection and data security from multicenters. It might be leveraged to collect multimodal EHR features from multicenters to train a large-scale model in a discrete distribution without collecting patients' EHR directly.

5.3 Explore More Ways of Interaction Between Modalities

There are still many limitations in the fusion methods of multimodal data. This issue is also a major direction that needs attention in future research. Most of the current research uses methods of direct concatenation to fuse multimodal data, either from the data or embedding level. This method is easy to implement, but the representation gap of different types of data is ignored. For example, embeddings trained with unstructured data are quite different from those trained with structured data in the semantic level, i.e. the semantic granularity is different [79]. Future research on the fusion strategy of multimodal data should find more ways to align the representation level of different modalities of data. Current works have tried different solutions, but a consensus on a widely accepted strategy for multimodal interaction, especially in the fusion method of structured and unstructured data, has not been retained yet. The interaction strategies of multimodal methods using different types of data, such as interaction of image data [80], structured data and text data, may be worth exploration and adoption among each other.

5.4 How and How Much Pretrained Models Can Help?

Pretrained models have been proved helpful in many natural language processing [81] as well as multimodal classification tasks (e.g. integrating image and text) [82]. Using pretrained models, comprehensive contextual information for both different modalities and their interactions could be learned in a self-supervised way [83] or with minimum supervisions [84]. For EHR mining, however, the explorations on multimodal data that contain both structured and unstructured text are limited. [71] is one representative study in this paradigm but it only applies shallow embedding techniques and fails to encode deeper contextual information. [85] is a pioneer study that pretrains with structured and unstructured data together using BERT, but it only uses the diagnosis information as the structured modality. Adopting more techniques from the general multimodal pretraining (e.g. VideoBERT [86]) or treating it as a machine translation problem [87] might be ways for further exploration.

6   Conclusions

This review summarizes current advances in multimodal EHR studies using both structured and unstructured free-text EHR data with conventional ML and DL techniques. We proposed interaction strategies, a new taxonomy targeted to the combination of structured and free-text EHR data. Our finding suggests that there is a growing interest in the modeling of multimodal EHR, but most studies combine the modalities with relatively simple strategies, which despite being shown to be effective, might not fully exploit the rich information embedded in these modalities. We acknowledge that there are still limitations with this review such as the limitation in the coverage of queried papers and included algorithms. As this is a fast-growing field and new models are constantly being developed, there might exist studies that fall outside of our definition of strategies or use a combination of these strategies. Nonetheless, we believe that the development of this field will give rise to more comprehensive EHR analysis and will be of great support to the clinical decision-making process.

Authors' Contributions. YX and ZYL conceived the study. ZYL designed search method, analyzed model aspect of included papers, and drafted most parts of the manuscript. JQZ participated in study design, analyzed task aspect of included papers, and drafted Task section. YSH analyzed cohort aspect of included papers, and drafted Cohort section. XRZ contributed to future direction, YX supervised the research, provided feedback to the proposed taxonomy, contributed to future direction, and critically revised the manuscript. GL participated in manuscript review. All authors provided feedback and approved the final version of the manuscript.

Funding. The paper is supported by the grant 62106115 from Natural Science Foundation of China.

References

1. Jha, A.K., DesRoches, C.M., Campbell, E.G., et al.: Use of electronic health records in U.S. hospitals, vol. 360, pp. 1628–1638 (2009). https://doi.org/10.1056/NEJMsa0900592
2. Rosenbloom, S.T., et al.: Data from clinical notes: a perspective on the tension between structure and flexible documentation. J. Am. Med. Inform. Assoc. JAMIA **18**, 181–186 (2011). https://doi.org/10.1136/JAMIA.2010.007237
3. Fox, K.M., et al.: Accuracy of medical records in hip fracture. J. Am. Geriatr. Soc. **46**, 745–750 (1998). https://doi.org/10.1111/J.1532-5415.1998.TB03810.X
4. Jensen, P.B., Jensen, L.J., Brunak, S.: Mining electronic health records: towards better research applications and clinical care. Nat. Rev. Genet. **13**(6), 395–405 (2012). https://doi.org/10.1038/nrg3208
5. Häyrinen, K., Saranto, K., Nykänen, P.: Definition, structure, content, use and impacts of electronic health records: a review of the research literature. Int. J. Med. Inform. **77**, 291–304 (2008). https://doi.org/10.1016/J.IJMEDINF.2007.09.001
6. Segura-Bedmar, I., Martínez, P., de Pablo-Sánchez, C.: Using a shallow linguistic kernel for drug–drug interaction extraction. J. Biomed. Inform. **44**, 789–804 (2011). https://doi.org/10.1016/J.JBI.2011.04.005
7. Rajkomar, A., Oren, E., Chen, K., et al.: Scalable and accurate deep learning with electronic health records. npj Digit. Med. **1**(1), 1–10 (2018). https://doi.org/10.1038/s41746-018-0029-1
8. Wang, Z., Yu, G., Kang, Y., et al.: Breast tumor detection in digital mammography based on extreme learning machine. Neurocomputing **128**, 175–184 (2014). https://doi.org/10.1016/J.NEUCOM.2013.05.053
9. Shivade, C., Raghavan, P., Fosler-Lussier, E., et al.: A review of approaches to identifying patient phenotype cohorts using electronic health records. J. Am. Med. Inform. Assoc. JAMIA **21**, 221 (2014). https://doi.org/10.1136/AMIAJNL-2013-001935
10. Hersh, W.R., et al.: Caveats for the use of operational electronic health record data in comparative effectiveness research. Med. Care **51** (2013). https://doi.org/10.1097/MLR.0B013E31829B1DBD

11. Birman-Deych, E., et al.: Accuracy of ICD-9-CM codes for identifying cardiovascular and stroke risk factors. Med. Care **43**, 480–485 (2005). https://doi.org/10.1097/01.MLR.000016 041739497.A9

12. Ford, E., Carroll, J.A., Smith, H.E., et al.: Extracting information from the text of electronic medical records to improve case detection: a systematic review. J. Am. Med. Inform. Assoc. **23**, 1007–1015 (2016). https://doi.org/10.1093/JAMIA/OCV180

13. Shickel, B., et al.: Deep EHR: a survey of recent advances in deep learning techniques for electronic health record (EHR) analysis. IEEE J. Biomed. Health Inform. **22**, 1589–1604 (2018). https://doi.org/10.1109/JBHI.2017.2767063

14. Xiao, C., Choi, E., Sun, J.: Opportunities and challenges in developing deep learning models using electronic health records data: a systematic review. J. Am. Med. Inform. Assoc. **25**, 1419–1428 (2018). https://doi.org/10.1093/JAMIA/OCY068

15. Si, Y., Du, J., Li, Z., et al.: Deep representation learning of patient data from electronic health records (EHR): a systematic review. J. Biomed. Inform. **115** (2021).https://doi.org/10.1016/ J.JBI.2020.103671

16. Zeng, Z., Deng, Y., Li, X., et al.: Natural language processing for EHR-based computational phenotyping. IEEE/ACM Trans. Comput. Biol. Bioinf. **16**, 139–153 (2019). https://doi.org/ 10.1109/TCBB.2018.2849968

17. Sheikhalishahi, S., Miotto, R., Dudley, J.T., et al.: Natural language processing of clinical notes on chronic diseases: systematic review. JMIR Med. Inform. **7** (2019). https://doi.org/ 10.2196/12239

18. Huang, S.-C., Pareek, A., Seyyedi, S., et al.: Fusion of medical imaging and electronic health records using deep learning: a systematic review and implementation guidelines. npj Digit. Med. **3**(1), 1–9 (2020). https://doi.org/10.1038/s41746-020-00341-z

19. Murray, S.G., Avati, A., Schmajuk, G., et al.: Automated and flexible identification of complex disease: building a model for systemic lupus erythematosus using noisy labeling. J. Am. Med. Inform. Assoc. **26**, 61–65 (2019). https://doi.org/10.1093/JAMIA/OCY154

20. Ananthakrishnan, A.N., Cai, T., Savova, G., et al.: Improving case definition of Crohn' s disease and ulcerative colitis in electronic medical records using natural language processing: a novel informatics approach. Inflamm. Bowel Dis. **19**, 1411–1420 (2013). https://doi.org/10. 1097/MIB.0B013E31828133FD

21. Teixeira, P.L., Wei, W.-Q., Cronin, R.M., et al.: Evaluating electronic health record data sources and algorithmic approaches to identify hypertensive individuals. J. Am. Med. Inform. Assoc. JAMIA **24**, 162 (2017). https://doi.org/10.1093/JAMIA/OCW071

22. Mugisha, C., Paik, I.: Pneumonia outcome prediction using structured and unstructured data from EHR. In: 2020 IEEE International Conference on Bioinformatics and Biomedicine (BIBM), 2640–2646 (2020). https://doi.org/10.1109/BIBM49941.2020.9312987

23. Jiang, H., Li, Y., Zeng, X., et al.: Exploring fever of unknown origin intelligent diagnosis based on clinical data: Model Dev. Valid. JMIR Med. Inform. **8** (2020). https://doi.org/10. 2196/24375

24. Afzal, Z., Engelkes, M., Verhamme, K.M.C., et al.: Automatic generation of case-detection algorithms to identify children with asthma from large electronic health record databases. Pharmacoepidemiol. Drug Saf. **22**, 826–833 (2013). https://doi.org/10.1002/PDS.3438

25. Henriksson, A., Zhao, J., Dalianis, H., et al.: Ensembles of randomized trees using diverse distributed representations of clinical events. BMC Med. Inform. Decis. Mak. **16** (2016). https://doi.org/10.1186/S12911-016-0309-0

26. Makino, M., Yoshimoto, R., Ono, M., et al.: Artificial intelligence predicts the progression of diabetic kidney disease using big data machine learning. Sci. Rep. **9**(1), 1–9 (2019). https:// doi.org/10.1038/s41598-019-48263-5

27. Tou, H., Yao, L., Wei, Z.: Automatic infection detection based on electronic medical records. In: 2017 IEEE International Conference on Bioinformatics and Biomedicine (BIBM), pp. 1684–1687 (2017). https://doi.org/10.1109/BIBM.2017.8217913

28. Zhang, D., Yin, C., Zeng, J., et al.: Combining structured and unstructured data for predictive models: a deep learning approach. BMC Med. Inform. Decis. Mak. **20** (2020). https://doi.org/10.1186/S12911-020-01297-6

29. Hu, S.Y., Santus, E., Forsyth, A.W., et al.: Can machine learning improve patient selection for cardiac resynchronization therapy? PLoS ONE **14** (2019). https://doi.org/10.1371/JOURNAL.PONE.0222397

30. Landi, I., Glicksberg, B.S., Lee, H.C., et al.: Deep representation learning of electronic health records to unlock patient stratification at scale. npj Digit. Med. **3** (2020). https://doi.org/10.1038/S41746-020-0301-Z

31. Liu, J., Zhang, Z., Razavian, N.: Deep EHR: chronic disease prediction using medical notes, pp. 440–464 (2018). http://proceedings.mlr.press/v85/liu18b.html. Accessed 13 July 2021

32. Johnson, A.E., et al.: MIMIC-III, a freely accessible critical care database. Sci. Data **3** (2016). https://doi.org/10.1038/SDATA.2016.35

33. Dm, R., Jm, P., Ma, B., et al.: Development of a large-scale de-identified DNA biobank to enable personalized medicine. Clin. Pharmacol. Ther. **84**, 362–369 (2008). https://doi.org/10.1038/CLPT.2008.89

34. Miotto, R., Li, L., Kidd, B.A., et al.: Deep patient: an unsupervised representation to predict the future of patients from the electronic health records. Sci. Rep. **6** (2016). https://doi.org/10.1038/SREP26094

35. Uzuner, Ö., Stubbs, A.: Practical applications for natural language processing in clinical research: the 2014 i2b2/UTHealth shared tasks. J. Biomed. Inform. **58**, S1 (2015). https://doi.org/10.1016/J.JBI.2015.10.007

36. Spasic, I., Nenadic, G.: Clinical text data in machine learning: systematic review. JMIR Med. Inform. **8** (2020). https://doi.org/10.2196/17984

37. Gultepe, E., Green, J.P., Nguyen, H., et al.: From vital signs to clinical outcomes for patients with sepsis: a machine learning basis for a clinical decision support system. J. Am. Med. Inform. Assoc. **21**, 315–325 (2014)

38. Zhao, J., Henriksson, A., Asker, L., et al.: Predictive modeling of structured electronic health records for adverse drug event detection. BMC Med. Inform. Decis. Mak. **15** (2015). https://doi.org/10.1186/1472-6947-15-S4-S1

39. Payrovnaziri, S.N., Barrett, L.A., Bis, D., et al.: Enhancing prediction models for one-year mortality in patients with acute myocardial infarction and post myocardial infarction syndrome. Stud. Health Technol. Inform. **264**, 273–277 (2019). https://doi.org/10.3233/SHTI190226

40. Nunes, A.P., et al.: Assessing occurrence of hypoglycemia and its severity from electronic health records of patients with type 2 diabetes mellitus. Diabetes Res. Clin. Pract. **121**, 192–203 (2016). https://doi.org/10.1016/J.DIABRES.2016.09.012

41. Meng, Y., Speier, W., Ong, M., et al.: HCET: hierarchical clinical embedding with topic modeling on electronic health records for predicting future depression. IEEE J. Biomed. Health Inform. **25**, 1265–1272 (2021). https://doi.org/10.1109/JBHI.2020.3004072

42. Xu, Z., Chou, J., Zhang, X.S., et al.: Identifying sub-phenotypes of acute kidney injury using structured and unstructured electronic health record data with memory networks. J. Biomed. Inform. **102** (2020). https://doi.org/10.1016/J.JBI.2019.103361

43. Amrollahi, F., Shashikumar, S.P., Razmi, F., et al.: Contextual embeddings from clinical notes improves prediction of sepsis. In: AMIA Annual Symposium Proceedings, pp. 197–202 (2020). 197./pmc/articles/PMC8075484/. Accessed 13 July 2021

44. Zeng, Z., et al.: Identifying breast cancer distant recurrences from electronic health records using machine learning. J. Healthc. Inform. Res. **3**(3), 283–299 (2019). https://doi.org/10.1007/s41666-019-00046-3

45. Zhang, X., Xiao, C., Glass, L.M., et al.: DeepEnroll: patient-trial matching with deep embedding and entailment prediction. In: Proceedings of the Web Conference 2020, pp. 1029–1037. Association for Computing Machinery, New York (2020). https://doi.org/10.1145/3366423.3380181

46. Xu, H., Fu, Z., Shah, A., et al.: Extracting and integrating data from entire electronic health records for detecting colorectal cancer cases. In: AMIA Annual Symposium proceedings/AMIA Symposium AMIA Symposium, pp. 1564–1572 (2011)

47. Gustafson, E., Pacheco, J., Wehbe, F., et al.: A machine learning algorithm for identifying atopic dermatitis in adults from electronic health records. In: Proceedings - 2017 IEEE International Conference on Healthcare Informatics, ICHI 2017, pp. 83–90 (2017). https://doi.org/10.1109/ICHI.2017.31

48. Scheurwegs, E., Luyckx, K., Luyten, L., et al.: Data integration of structured and unstructured sources for assigning clinical codes to patient stays. J. Am. Med. Inform. Assoc. **23**, e11–e19 (2016). https://doi.org/10.1093/JAMIA/OCV115

49. Lin, C., Karlson, E.W., Canhao, H., et al.: Automatic prediction of rheumatoid arthritis disease activity from the electronic medical records. PLoS ONE **8** (2013)

50. Fodeh, S.J., Li, T., Jarad, H., et al.: Classification of patients with coronary microvascular dysfunction. IEEE/ACM Trans. Comput. Biol. Bioinform. **17**, 704–711 (2020). https://doi.org/10.1109/TCBB.2019.2914442

51. Chen, Y., Carroll, R.J., Hinz, E.R.M.P., et al. Applying active learning to high-throughput phenotyping algorithms for electronic health records data. J. Am. Med. Inform. Assoc. **20** (2013)

52. Zhao, D., Weng, C.: Combining PubMed knowledge and EHR data to develop a weighted Bayesian network for pancreatic cancer prediction. J. Biomed. Inform. **44**, 859 (2011). https://doi.org/10.1016/J.JBI.2011.05.004

53. LeCun, Y., Bengio, Y., Hinton, G.: Deep learning. Nature **521**(7553), 436–444 (2015). https://doi.org/10.1038/nature14539

54. Mikolov, T., Chen, K., Corrado, G., et al.: Efficient estimation of word representations in vector space. In: 1st International Conference on Learning Representations, ICLR 2013 - Workshop Track Proceedings, 16 January 2013. https://arxiv.org/abs/1301.3781v3. Accessed 13 Aug 2021

55. Devlin, J., Chang, M.-W., Lee, K., et al.: BERT: pre-training of deep bidirectional transformers for language understanding. In: NAACL HLT 2019 - 2019 Conference of the North American Chapter of the Association for Computational Linguistics: Human Language Technologies - Proceedings of the Conference, vol. 1, pp. 4171–4186 (2018). https://arxiv.org/abs/1810.04805v2. Accessed 13 Aug 2021

56. Yin, W., Kann, K., Yu, M., et al.: Comparative study of CNN and RNN for natural language processing, 7 February 2017. https://arxiv.org/abs/1702.01923v1. Accessed 13 July 2021

57. Hochreiter, S., Schmidhuber, J.: Long short-term memory. Neural Comput. **9**, 1735–1780 (1997). https://doi.org/10.1162/NECO.1997.9.8.1735

58. Huang, K., Altosaar, J., Ranganath, R.: ClinicalBERT: modeling clinical notes and predicting hospital readmission, 10 April 2019. https://arxiv.org/abs/1904.05342v3. Accessed 13 July 2021

59. Darabi, S., Kachuee, M., Fazeli, S., et al.: TAPER: time-aware patient EHR representation. IEEE J. Biomed. Health Inform. **24**, 3268–3275 (2020). https://doi.org/10.1109/JBHI.2020.2984931

60. Lee, D., Jiang, X., Yu, H.: Harmonized representation learning on dynamic EHR graphs. J. Biomed. Inform. **106** (2020). https://doi.org/10.1016/J.JBI.2020.103426

61. Wang, L., Sha, L., Lakin, J.R., et al.: Development and validation of a deep learning algorithm for mortality prediction in selecting patients with dementia for earlier palliative care interventions. JAMA Netw. Open **2**, e196972–e196972 (2019). https://doi.org/10.1001/JAMANETWORKOPEN.2019.6972

62. Liao, K.P., Cai, T., Gainer, V., et al.: Electronic medical records for discovery research in rheumatoid arthritis. Arthritis Care Res. **62**, 1120–1127 (2010)

63. Henriksson, A., Zhao, J., Boström, H., et al.: Modeling electronic health records in ensembles of semantic spaces for adverse drug event detection. In: 2015 IEEE International Conference on Bioinformatics and Biomedicine (BIBM), pp. 343–350 (2015). https://doi.org/10.1109/BIBM.2015.7359705

64. Beeksma, M., Verberne, S., van den Bosch, A., et al.: Predicting life expectancy with a long short-term memory recurrent neural network using electronic medical records. BMC Med. Inform. Decis. Mak. **19** (2019). https://doi.org/10.1186/S12911-019-0775-2

65. Liu, R., Greenstein, J.L., Sarma, S.V., et al.: Natural language processing of clinical notes for improved early prediction of septic shock in the ICU. In: 2019 41st Annual International Conference of the IEEE Engineering in Medicine and Biology Society (EMBC), pp. 6103–6108 (2019). https://doi.org/10.1109/EMBC.2019.8857819

66. Bardak, B., Tan, M.: Improving clinical outcome predictions using convolution over medical entities with multimodal learning. Artif. Intell. Med. **117** (2021). https://doi.org/10.1016/J.ARTMED.2021.102112

67. Bagheri, A., Groenhof, T.K.J., Veldhuis, W.B., et al.: Multimodal learning for cardiovascular risk prediction using EHR data. In: Proceedings of the 11th ACM International Conference on Bioinformatics, Computational Biology and Health Informatics. Association for Computing Machinery, New York (2020). https://doi.org/10.1145/3388440.3414924

68. Xie, X., Xiong, Y., Yu, P.S., et al.: EHR coding with multi-scale feature attention and structured knowledge graph propagation. In: Proceedings of the 28th ACM International Conference on Information and Knowledge Management, pp. 649–658. Association for Computing Machinery, New York (2019). https://doi.org/10.1145/3357384.3357897

69. Shin, B., Hogan, J., Adams, A.B., et al.: Multimodal ensemble approach to incorporate various types of clinical notes for predicting readmission. In: 2019 IEEE EMBS International Conference on Biomedical & Health Informatics (BHI), pp. 1–4 (2019). https://doi.org/10.1109/BHI.2019.8834640

70. Xu, K., Lam, M., Pang, J., et al.: Multimodal machine learning for automated ICD coding. In: Proceedings of Machine Learning Research, vol. 106, pp. 197–215 (2019). http://proceedings.mlr.press/v106/xu19a.html. Accessed 13 July 2021

71. Bai, T., Chanda, A.K., Egleston, B.L., et al.: EHR phenotyping via jointly embedding medical concepts and words into a unified vector space. BMC Med. Inform. Decis. Mak. **18** (2018). https://doi.org/10.1186/S12911-018-0672-0

72. Blei, D.M., Ng, A.Y., Jordan, M.I.: Latent Dirichlet allocation. J. Mach. Learn. Res. **3**, 993–1022 (2003). https://doi.org/10.1016/b978-0-12-411519-4.00006-9

73. Savova, G.K., Masanz, J.J., Ogren, P.V., et al.: Mayo clinical text analysis and knowledge extraction system (cTAKES): architecture, component evaluation and applications. J. Am. Med. Inform. Assoc. JAMIA **17**, 507 (2010). https://doi.org/10.1136/JAMIA.2009.001560

74. Aronson, A.R.: Effective mapping of biomedical text to the UMLS metathesaurus: the MetaMap program. In: Proceedings AMIA Symposium, pp. 17–21 (2001). https://pubmed.ncbi.nlm.nih.gov/11825149/. Accessed 13 Aug 2021

75. Denny, J.C., Irani, P.R., Wehbe, F.H., et al.: The KnowledgeMap project: development of a concept-based medical school curriculum database. In: AMIA Annual Symposium Proceedings, p. 195 (2003). 195./pmc/articles/PMC1480333/. Accessed 13 Aug 2021

76. Zeng, Q.T., Goryachev, S., Weiss, S., et al.: Extracting principal diagnosis, co-morbidity and smoking status for asthma research: evaluation of a natural language processing system. BMC Med. Inform. Decis. Mak. **6**(1), 1–9 (2006).https://doi.org/10.1186/1472-6947-6-30

77. Vaswani, A., Shazeer, N., Parmar, N., et al.: Attention is all you need. In: Advances in Neural Information Processing Systems, December 2017, pp. 5999–6009. https://arxiv.org/abs/1706.03762v5. Accessed 4 Sept 2021

78. Venugopalan, J., Tong, L., Hassanzadeh, H.R., et al.: Multimodal deep learning models for early detection of Alzheimer' s disease stage. Sci. Rep. **11**(1), 1–13 (2021). https://doi.org/10.1038/s41598-020-74399-w

79. Rasmy, L., Xiang, Y., Xie, Z., et al.: Med-BERT: pretrained contextualized embeddings on large-scale structured electronic health records for disease prediction. npj Digit. Med. **4**(1), 1–13 (2021). https://doi.org/10.1038/s41746-021-00455-y

80. Zhang, X., Chou, J., Liang, J., et al.: Data-driven subtyping of Parkinson' s disease using longitudinal clinical records: a cohort study. Sci. Rep. **9**(1), 1–12 (2019). https://doi.org/10.1038/s41598-018-37545-z

81. Qiu, X., Sun, T., Xu, Y., Shao, Y., Dai, N., Huang, X.: Pre-trained models for natural language processing: a survey. Sci. China Technol. Sci. **63**(10), 1872–1897 (2020). https://doi.org/10.1007/s11431-020-1647-3

82. Li, Y., Wang, H., Luo, Y.: A comparison of pre-trained vision-and-language models for multimodal representation learning across medical images and reports. In: Proceedings - 2020 IEEE International Conference on Bioinformatics and Biomedicine, BIBM, pp. 1999–2004 (2020). https://doi.org/10.1109/BIBM49941.2020.9313289

83. Akbari, H., Yuan, L., Qian, R., et al.: VATT: transformers for multimodal self-supervised learning from raw video, audio and text, 22 April 2021. https://arxiv.org/abs/2104.11178v1. Accessed 14 July 2021

84. Bouritsas, G., Koutras, P., Zlatintsi, A., et al.: Multimodal visual concept learning with weakly supervised techniques. In: Proceedings of the IEEE Conference on Computer Vision and Pattern Recognition (CVPR), pp. 4914–4923 (2018)

85. Shang, J., Ma, T., Xiao, C., et al.: Pre-training of graph augmented transformers for medication recommendation. In: IJCAI International Joint Conference on Artificial Intelligence, August 2019, pp. 5953–5959. https://arxiv.org/abs/1906.00346v2. Accessed 12 Sept 2021

86. Sun, C., Myers, A., Vondrick, C., et al.: VideoBERT: a joint model for video and language representation learning. In: Proceedings of the IEEE International Conference on Computer Vision, October 2019, pp. 7463 – 7472. https://arxiv.org/abs/1904.01766v2. Accessed 14 July 2021

87. Bahdanau, D., Cho, K., Bengio, Y.: Neural machine translation by jointly learning to align and translate. In: 3rd International Conference on Learning Representations, ICLR 2015 - Conference Track Proceedings, 1 September 2014. https://arxiv.org/abs/1409.0473v7. Accessed 4 Sept 2021

88. Li, T., Sahu, A.K., Talwalkar, A., et al.: federated learning: challenges, methods, and future directions. IEEE Signal Process. Mag. **37**, 50–60 (2020). https://doi.org/10.1109/MSP.2020.2975749

89. DeLisle, S., Kim, B., Deepak, J., et al.: Using the electronic medical record to identify communityacquired pneumonia: toward a replicable automated strategy. PLoS ONE **8**(8), e70944 (2013)

An End-to-End Knowledge Graph Based Question Answering Approach for COVID-19

Yinbo Qiao, Zhihao Yang[✉], Hongfei Lin, and Jian Wang

Dalian University of Technology, Dalian 116024, China
`yinboqiao@mail.dlut.edu.cn`, {`yangzh,hflin,wangjian`}`@dlut.edu.cn`

Abstract. Question Answering based on Knowledge Graph (KG) has emerged as a popular research area in general domain. However, few works focus on the COVID-19 kg-based question answering, which is very valuable for biomedical domain. In addition, existing question answering methods rely on knowledge embedding models to represent knowledge (i.e., entities and questions), but the relations between entities are neglected. In this paper, we construct a COVID-19 knowledge graph and propose an end-to-end knowledge graph question answering approach that can utilize relation information to improve the performance. Experimental result shows that the effectiveness of our approach on the COVID-19 knowledge graph question answering. Our code and data are available at https://github.com/CHNcreater/COVID-19-KGQA.

Keywords: COVID-19 · Knowledge graph · Knowledge graph embedding

1 Introduction

A knowledge graph is a structured database which contains a collection of factoids with the format of <subject, relation, object>. Currently, several large-scale knowledge graphs have been constructed, such as Freebase [1], DBPedia [2] and Yago [3], which can be used to serve question answering tasks. One important application of these knowledge graphs is question answering and knowledge graph based question answering (KGQA) has become an important research area. Based on available KGs, KGQA aims to understand the natural language (NL) questions asked by users and retrieve the answer entities in KGs. At present, several works have been proposed on publicly available KG [4, 5]. However, few works pay attention to COVID-19 knowledge graph based question answering. COVID-19 is severe and has caused millions of deaths around the world. Although a lot of information available on COVID-19, the information is not well organized and specialized for the general public. Therefore, we constructed a COVID-19KG and propose a COVID-19 question answering approach to satisfy the needs of people.

Early works on KGQA [6–8] focus on answering simple questions, which only need a single triplet to support. For example, "what disease does coronavirus cause?" is a simple query that can be answered by the fact "coronavirus, cause, COVID-19". Recently, the complex question over KGs, which often contains multiple subjects and relations,

B. Tang et al. (Eds.): CHIP 2022, CCIS 1772, pp. 156–169, 2023.
https://doi.org/10.1007/978-981-19-9865-2_11

attracts more attention than the simple question. The complex question answering system needs to reason over multiple edges of the KG to infer the right answer entities. Complex question methods can be divided into two mainstream approaches, i.e., SP-based methods and IR-based methods [9]. The SP-based approach focuses on generating a logical form of question and then executing it against the KGs and searching for the final answers. Another line of works is IR-based methods. The latter methods construct a subgraph related to the given question and rank the candidate entities in the extracted subgraph based on their relevance to the question. Overall, the SP-based methods are more interpretable, where we can observe all intermediate reasoning steps and how the methods find the final answer. But they heavily depend on the reliable design of logic form and path reasoning. Moreover, SP-based methods require experts to analyze question semantically or syntactically and formulate some logic templates which can be execute against KGs to generate answer. These problems become the bottleneck of SP-based methods and make their models difficult to train. On the contrary, IR-based methods directly retrieve answers from KGs. They first extract a subgraph for each question and then utilize encoding module to embed questions into vector. Next, vector-based reasoning module conducts semantic matching over the subgraph. Finally, answer ranking module is deployed to choose the answer. Most calculations are based on vectors, and therefore IR-based methods fit into end-to-end training and are easy to train.

Recently, some recent methods have been proposed for KGQA tasks [5, 10–13]. However, most of the methods suffer from the inevitable incompleteness problems of knowledge graph, which severely affects the performance of the question answering system [10]. To solve this problem Sun et al. [5, 11] proposed GRAFT-Net to fuse Wikipedia as an external text corpus. Specifically, Sun et al. [5] constructed a question-specific subgraph from KG and then augmented it with a text corpus consisted of documents, but the identification and selection of relevant text documents is a challenge that limits the performance of the method. Moreover, this method also has limitation in neighborhood size of subgraph, which causes the right answer cannot be included in the subgraph. Xiong et al. [12] and Han et al. [13] proposed to fuse extra text representation information into entities representation to alleviate the incompleteness of knowledge graph. In particular, they encoded the sentences and entities based on the question, then supplemented the entities representations with sentences representations. In addition, they also took advantage of the knowledge graph embedding to address the sparsity problem of KGs. Saxena et al. [14] capitalized the knowledge graph embedding method to enrich the representations of entities and then calculates the scores of the candidate entities. Nevertheless, their method neglects the relation path information, failing to match the right entities well.

To address the above challenges, we apply the knowledge graph embedding and popular end-to-end training to the COVID-19 knowledge graph question answering model. Our contributions can be summarized as follows.

- Due to the lack of a COVID-19 knowledge graph, we constructed a knowledge base about COVID-19 via NER (Named Entity Recognition) and Relation Extraction algorithms from PubMed biomedical texts.
- We created a COVID-19 question answering dataset based on the COVID-19 knowledge graph through question templates and rules.

- We utilized the knowledge graph embedding to alleviate the incompleteness of KGs. Experimental results prove the method is effective for the COVID-19 KGQA task and achieves the state-of-the-art result on COVID-19 question answering dataset.

2 Background

2.1 Task Definition

The KGQA task in this work aims to answer a natural language question over knowledge graph triples $\mathcal{K} = \{(h, r, t)|h \in \mathcal{E}, r \in \mathcal{R}\}$, where $\mathcal{E}$ and $\mathcal{R}$ is the set of entities and relations respectively. Given a natural language question, like Saxena et al. [14], we encode the natural language question into a vector. Taking into account the incompleteness of the knowledge graph, knowledge graph embedding is more suitable for the COVID-19KG question answering. At first, we embed the entities and relations of COVID-19 knowledge graph into vectors. Subsequently, the model represents the question into continuous vector space and then tries to retrieve answer entities from candidate entities.

2.2 Knowledge Graph

A knowledge graph is a structured database that contains a set of triples such that (h, r, t), where h, t represent entities and r represent relationships between h and t, respectively. We constructed a COVID-19 knowledge graph as the knowledge source of our QA method. We call this knowledge graph the self-constructed COVID-19 knowledge graph (COVID-19KG).

The data of COVID-19KG is extracted from a total of 23,373 full texts downloaded from PubMed using the query of "COVID-19" [All Fields] OR "COVID-2019" [All Fields] OR "severe acute respiratory syndrome coronavirus 2" [Supplementary Concept] OR "severe acute respiratory syndrome coronavirus 2" [All Fields] OR "2019-nCoV" [All Fields] OR "SARS-CoV-2" [All Fields] OR "2019nCoV" [All Fields] OR (("Wuhan"[All Fields] AND ("coronavirus" [MeSH Terms] OR "coronavirus" [All Fields])) AND (2019/12[PDAT] OR 2020/06[PDAT])) AND "loattrfree full text"). We trained the name entity recognition and relation extraction models, then used them to extract the KG triples. The model details will be introduced in section experiments.

2.3 Knowledge Graph Embedding

The knowledge graph is a multi-relational directed graph composed of entities (the nodes of the graph) and relations (the edges of the graph). Although this kind of structured data can store the KG triples, these symbolic triples are difficult to calculate directly in deep learning models. To address this issue, a new direction known as Knowledge Graph Embedding (KGE) has been proposed. The main idea is to embed the components of KGs, such as entities and relations, into continuous vector space. For each $e \in \mathcal{E}$ and $r \in \mathcal{R}$, we use knowledge graph embedding (KGE) methods to generate $\mathcal{V}_e \in \mathbb{R}^{d_e}$ and $\mathcal{V}_r \in \mathbb{R}^{d_r}$, where $\mathcal{V}_e$ and $\mathcal{V}_r$ are d_e and d_r dimensional vector representation respectively. The KGE models measure all triples (h, r, t) to make sure every correct triple score $\phi(h, r, t) > 0$ and wrong triple score $\phi(h', r', t') < 0$, where $(h, r, t) \in \mathcal{K}$ and $(h', r', t') \notin \mathcal{K}$. Currently, a range of KGE models have been proposed to train knowledge graph [9], such as ComplEx, RESCAL, DistMult, SimplE and TuckER.

3   Method

In this section, we provide the problem statement and the model overview. Subsequently, we describe in detail the main modules of our method and explain the implementation details.

3.1   Problem Statement

Let $\mathcal{K} \subseteq \mathcal{E} \times \mathcal{R} \times \mathcal{E}$ be the set of triplets, where $\mathcal{E}$ and $\mathcal{R}$ is the set of entities and relations respectively. Given a natural language question q and a top entity $e \in \mathcal{E}$ which is marked in the question, the KGQA aims to understand the question and extract the correct answer entity e_{answer} from KG. The overall framework is shown in Fig. 2.

3.2   Information Extraction Model Overview

Figure 1 depicts the information extraction model, which involves three major modules, i.e., name entity recognition, binary relation extraction and relation word extraction.

1) Name Entity Recognition. We use the BERT-CRF [31] to acquire entities from biomedical literature. This NER module can extract eight kinds of entities, i.e., drug, disease, protein, DNA, RNA, cell, phenotype and mutation. The BERT-CRF model is trained on CDR [22] and NLPBA [23] dataset to recognize entities. To further improve the accuracy and performance of NER, we also deploy the dictionary-based method to recognize the entities which BERT-CRF cannot extract. For evaluation, we split the training corpus into training, develop and test sets. Like previous work

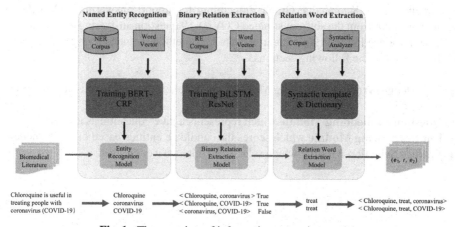

Fig. 1. The overview of information extraction model.

on NER [31], we adopt F1 value as evaluation metrics. Finally, the F1 value of our name entity recognition can reach 85% (http://www.medicalqa.xyz/precision_med icine/index.html is published as a demo).

2) Binary Relation Extraction. The Binary Relation Extraction (BRE) model is designed to judge whether the recognized entities have semantic relations. As shown in Fig. 1, the BRE model predict that the entity Chloroquine have semantic relation with the entity coronavirus. The BRE model is trained on the training part of the dataset.
3) Relation Word Extraction. The relation word extraction module further uses syntactic rules to extract specific relation trigger words from entity pairs with relations.

We performed the data cleaning and deduplication on the triples in the knowledge graph to make sure that one entity corresponds to only one ID. The statistics of COVID-19KG are showed in Table 1. It contains about 11K entities, 8K relationships, and 120K facts (if not stated otherwise, we use COVID-19KG to represent the COVID-19 knowledge graph).

Table 1. The statistics of COVID-19KG.

COVID-19KG	
Entities	11,264
Relationships	8,038
Triples	123,190

3.3 Question Answering Method Overview

Our method uses Knowledge Graph Embedding to support answering a COVID-19 related question from the self-constructed COVID-19 question answering dataset which will be introduced in the Experiment section. Our method includes four parts and will be introduced in the following sections.

- **Knowledge Graph Embedding Module** which generates representations of entities and relations.
- **Question Embedding Module** which represents a given question as a vector.
- **Entities Scoring Module** which scores the candidate entities based on KGE model.
- **Entities Selection Module** which selects the final answer entities.

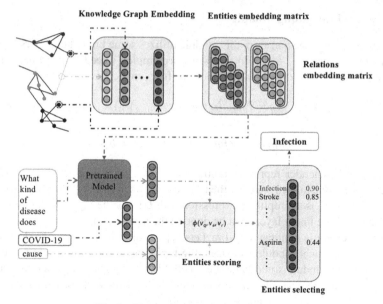

Fig. 2. The model for COVID-19KGQA.

3.4 Knowledge Graph Embedding Module

We utilize different types of KGE models to embed entities and relations of COVID-19KG into vectors. To get embedding of COVID-19KG, we use a tool called LibKGE [24] to exploit different KGE models. Then we select the KGE model which works best on the valid set and evaluate it on the test set. In addition, we trained five popular KGE models, which are ComplEx, RESCAL, DistMult, SimplE and TuckER. As regards evaluation metrics, we employ hit@1 for the model evaluation.

These KGE methods are trained for all entities and relations to get their representations in the fixed dimension vector. Moreover, the trained embeddings are used to initialize the entities embedding and relations embedding in pretrained model which embeds the questions into vectors. We take the ComplEx model for example to introduce the KGE model.

Given $h, t \in \mathcal{E}$ and $r \in \mathcal{R}$, ComplEx model embeds entities and relations into vectors $v_h, v_r, v_t \in \mathbb{R}^d$. The score function is define as (1).

$$\phi(h, \mathrm{r}, \mathrm{t}) = \mathrm{Re}(\langle v_h, v_\mathrm{r}, v_\mathrm{t} \rangle) \tag{1}$$

$\phi(\cdot)$ is the scoring function of ComplEx. If $(h, r, t) \in \mathcal{K}$, $\phi(h, r, t) > 0$. Otherwise, $\phi(h, r, t) < 0$.

3.5 Question Embedding Module

Given a natural language question, this module utilizes some kind of encoders to embed questions into a vector $v_q \in \mathbb{R}^d$. In this work, we employ a feed-forward network that contains question embedding modules and four fully connected linear layers.

$$v_q = Encoder((w_1, w_2, \cdots, w_n)) \tag{2}$$

$$output = softmax(ReLU(v_q W + b)) \tag{3}$$

In this work, encoder represent pretrained model, such as BERT, BioBERT and RoBERTa. Using the hidden states of the first special token from pretrained models, i.e., [CLS]. Formula (3) is a simplified expression. $ReLU(\cdot)$ is the input for the next linear layer. The rest three linear layers can be done in the same manner.

The topic entity is annotated by brackets "[]" in question. Hence, we do not need to design an additional module to extract the topic entity and corresponding relation. We only need to conduct some heuristics methods to acquire them, such as syntactic parsing. Moreover, we can directly obtain their embedding vectors, which are $\mathcal{V}_q$ and $\mathcal{V}_r$, via COVID-19KG entities and relations embedding matrix.

3.6 Entities Scoring Module

Through the first two modules, we obtain the question vector representation v_q and embeddings of entities and relations. Then we define the candidate entities set as $\mathcal{A} = \{v_a | a \in \mathcal{E}\}$. Entities Scoring Module will learn a score function in a way as shown in formulas (4) and (5).

$$\phi(v_e, v_q + v_r, v_a) > 0 \forall a \in \mathcal{A} \tag{4}$$

$$\phi(v_e, v_q + v_r, v_{a'}) < 0 \forall a' \notin \mathcal{A} \tag{5}$$

$\phi(\cdot)$ is a scoring function depending on the KGE model used and a, a' are entities representations which are learned in Knowledge Graph Embedding step.

The aim of this module is to make the representation of question more related to triples (h, r, t) which can support answering the given question. Its another goal is to calculate the scores of all candidate entities. The model is trained by minimizing binary cross-entropy loss between scores and gold label, where 1 is for correct answer and 0 for wrong answer.

3.7 Entities Selection Module

After scoring all candidate entities, we can obtain the scores of every candidate entity. Since COVID-19KG is a relatively small knowledge graph, we simply select final entity with the highest score.

$$e_{answer} = arg \max_{a \in \mathcal{E}} \phi(v_e, v_q, v_a) \tag{6}$$

However, if the KG is large, we can exploit some heuristics to prune the candidate entities, which can significantly improve the performance of entities selection module. For example, we can calculate the similarity between relations and questions and then we only select the relations that scores higher than a threshold.

4 Experiments

In this section, we will introduce how the question answering dataset is constructed and then explain the experimental setup.

4.1 COVID-19KG

As shown in Table 1, COVID-19KG includes 11,264 entities, 8,038 relations, and 123,190 triples. As the knowledge source of question answering method, the quality of knowledge graph determines the performance of question answering task.

We evaluated the quality of COVID-19 knowledge graph from the following aspects.

1) Semantic accuracy. Semantic accuracy refers to the degree to which triplets correctly represent real-world phenomena. Considering the huge amount of triplets, we utilize random sampling to evaluate the semantic accuracy. After acquiring sampling data, we calculate the number of correct triplets via manual evaluation. The final accuracy is about 40%. The reason is that, confined to the complexity of natural language, automatically extracting entity relations to construct knowledge graph from the biomedical literature remains a challenging task, and it is difficult to achieve a satisfactory performance.

2) Population completeness. Overall integrity provides the percentage of all real entities of a particular type represented in the dataset. Considering the COVID-19KGQA dataset is generated from COVID-19 knowledge graph, the entities coverage is 100%. Similarly, by means of random sampling combined with manual evaluation, the proportion of real entities is about 80%.

3) Question answering task evaluation. In additional, we evaluated COVID-19KG through the question answering task. We embedded COVID-19KG into fixed dimension vectors and then used these vectors in our QA models. The KGE result is shown in Fig. 2 and the QA task result is shown in Table 3. Through analyzing the corresponding results, we can see that the quality of COVID-19KG can support COVID-19 question answering well.

4.2 Datasets

COVID-19QA Dataset: We introduce a new COVID-19 related QA dataset. Like MetaQA [18] dataset, we generate the question of the dataset from the limited number of question templates, which is a total of six kinds of "wh" question templates. Like WebQuestions [19] dataset, questions are mostly one-hop questions that include a small subgraph for each question. Our COVID-19QA dataset has some features as follows:

1) *One-hop question*: all questions in COVID-19QA are single-hop questions, which means only one single triple is involved.

2) *No noise on top entity*: we include the top entity in question by using "[]". For example, in the question, "what diseases could [Acute respiratory infections] cause?", the top entity is "Acute respiratory infections". Meanwhile, since there is no noise about the top entity, the top entity is easy to distinguish.

3) *Generated from text templates*: using crowded workers to rewrite and design questions is a laborious and cost-expensive task. Refer to the construction of MetaQA, we generate the questions by random sampling from question templates collections. All questions begin with "wh", which are "which" and "what".

4) *Based on COVID-19KG*: we construct the questions based on our self-constructed COVID-19 knowledge graph.

The COVID-19QA contains more than 200K questions for one-hop questions. We divide the COVID-19KGQA into training set and test set as shown in Table 2.

Table 2. COVID-19KGQA in this paper.

	Train	Test/Dev	KB	LF	NL
COVID-19KGQA	96,359	6.200	COVID-19KG	No	No

[a] LF denotes whether the dataset provides logic form. NL means whether the dataset is rewritten by human.

4.3 Baselines

We conducted experiments on COVID-19KGQA question answering dataset and employed three strong baselines. The first baseline is state-of-the-art models Embed-KGQA [14]. In addition, we changed the encoder component, such as BERT [25] and BioBERT [26], as the other two baselines methods. We compare with them under all settings. The Table 3 shows the result on COVID-19KGQA test set. As shown by results, our model performs the best.

4.4 Implementation Details

Firstly, we embedded entities and relations into vector representations. To get better performance of knowledge graph embedding, like Ruffinelli et al. [20], we utilized LibKGE [21] framework to train for all entities and relations.

LibKGE provides the best implements of the KGE models and is easy to use. In training process, we employed two knowledge graph settings, which are full COVID-19 knowledge graph and 50% COVID-19 knowledge graph, respectively. In experiments, we randomly remove half of triples to construct 50% COVID-19KG. We set the same configure file for the two knowledge graphs, such as max epochs, batch size and optimizer.

We implemented all models based on Pytorch [27]. With respect to pretrained models, such as Roberta [28], BERT and BioBERT, we utilized the corresponding models from Transformers library [29]. The entities and relations embedding dimension is set up to 200. In training process, we used Adam optimizer [30] to optimize the parameters and adopted the suggested hyper-parameters. The learning rate is set to 5e−3. For all the experiments, we choose the model which works best on test set. All experiments were conducted on GeForce RTX 3090 and TITAN Xp. The epoch number is set to 90 and early stop is set up 10.

4.5 Main Results

Following Saxena et al. [14], we evaluate the performance of QA methods using hit@1 score. Table 3 shows the results of the models on COVID-19KGQA question answering dataset.

From the results, we have the following three observations:

- Our framework outperforms the other methods and achieves the state-of-the-art performance. On COVID-19KGQA dataset, it achieves 1.3% improvement on hit@1 score over EmbedKGQA. This indicates that the relation information successfully incorporates relevant information to improve the performance.
- The hit@1 score with half knowledge graph setting have little gap with that of full knowledge graph setting.
- With the same setting, our method achieves a higher hit@1 score than the models which use BERT and BioBERT.

Table 3. Test result on COVID-19KGQA dataset.

Model	COVID-19KG (FULL)	COVID-19KF (50%)
EmbedKGQA [14]	0.277	0.282
EmbedWBERT	0.064	0.059
EmbedWBioBERT	0.075	0.072
(Ours method)	0.29	0.289

[b] Hit@1 of the three baseline models.

5 Analysis

5.1 Effect on Incompleteness of COVID-19KG

In experiments, we have two kind of knowledge graph settings which are full knowledge graph and 50% knowledge graph. The latter setting is to verify whether our method can address the incompleteness problem.

Our method utilizes the KGE to answer the question. It uses the top entity representation and question representation, which can capture the relations of all entities around the top entity. Unlike the other QA methods, our method can answer the question even if there is no direct path between the top entity and answer entity.

To verify the capability to address sparsity of knowledge graph, we design an experiment with 50% knowledge graph as shown in Table 3. According to the result, we found that the hit@1 of 50% knowledge graph is almost the same with that of full knowledge graph which shows that our method still works well for COVID-19 knowledge graph-based question answering even if the knowledge graph is sparse and incomplete.

5.2 Ablation Study

In addition, we study the impact of relation information on the model performance. Previous works ignored the relation embedding information in their models. However, the relation embedding does help model to capture more features of questions. To examine the effectiveness of relation embedding, we designed the ablation experiment. The result is shown in Table 4.

Without the relation part, we find that the performance of our method decreases by 0.5%. Table 4 shows the importance of incorporating relation information.

Table 4. Ablation study result.

Model	COVID-19KG (FULL)	COVID-19KG (50%)
w/o relation	0.282	0.277
w relation	0.285	0.282

5.3 Knowledge Graph Embedding Analysis

We select several popular knowledge graph embedding methods to represent COVID-19 knowledge graph. RuffinelliS et al. [20] argued that the choice of training strategy, hyperparameters and KGE models are very influential on model performance. We compared five types of KGE models, which are ComplEx, DistMult, RESCAL, SimplE and TuckER. In the training process, the hit@1 measure changes as shown in Fig. 3. The hit@1 is often used in knowledge graph embedding, which means the count of how many correct factoids (or triplets) are ranked in the top 1 position against a bunch of wrong ones.

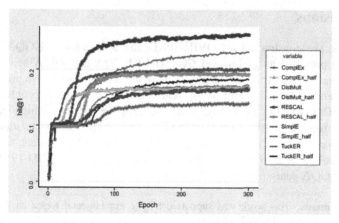

Fig. 3. Hit@1 curve of different KGE methods over COVID-19KG. The x axis represents the train epoch which is 300 epochs, and the y axis is the hit@1 index.

We found the RESCAL model achieve the best hit@1 score among the five models. To better verify the impact of KGE models, we design the following experiments. We choose the ComplEx and RESCAL models to verify the impact of different KGE models. The results are shown in Table 5.

Table 5. The KGE models.

Model	COVID-19KG (FULL)	COVID-19KG (50%)
w TuckER	0.285	0.282
w RESCAL	0.29	0.289

The experimental results show that the model which achieves higher hit@1 score would have better question answering performance.

5.4 Limitation Analysis

In this section, we analyze the limitation of QA method. We found the following reasons that damage the performance.

1) The lack of human rewritten. The questions are generated from very limited question templates, which causes a low diversity of problems.
2) Simple question structure. The questions start with "which" and "what", and the question structure is relatively simple.

6 Conclusions

In this work, we constructed a COVID-19KG and a COVID-19 KGQA dataset. In addition, we provided an end-to-end COVID-19 KGQA method. A self-constructed KG always has the incompleteness problems while recent works have proved knowledge graph embedding is useful to alleviate such incompleteness problem. To construct COVID-19KGQA, we utilize KGE and propose a model which incorporates relation information for the COVID-19KGQA task. Experimental results show our model achieves the best performance compared with the other models, which means the KGE method is also effective for the self-constructed COVID-19KG and the COVID-19KGQA dataset.

Acknowledgements. This work was supported by the Fundamental Research Funds for the Central Universities (No. DUT22ZD205).

References

1. Bollacker, K., Evans, C., Paritosh, P., Sturge, T., Taylor, J.: Freebase: a collaboratively created graph database for structuring human knowledge. In: Proceedings of the 2008 ACM SIGMOD International Conference on Management of Data (2008)
2. Lehmann, J., et al.: DBpedia–a large-scale, multilingual knowledge base extracted from wikipedia. Semantic Web **6**(2), 167–195 (2015)
3. Suchanek, F.M., Kasneci, G., Weikum, G.: Yago: a core of semantic knowledge. In: Proceedings of the 16th International Conference on World Wide Web (2007)
4. Zhang, Y., Dai, H., Kozareva, Z., Smola, A.J., Song, L.: Variational reasoning for question answering with knowledge graph. In: Thirty-Second AAAI Conference on Artificial Intelligence (2018)
5. Sun, H., Bedrax-Weiss, T., Cohen, W.W.: PullNet: open domain question answering with iterative retrieval on knowledge bases and text. arXiv preprint arXiv:1904.09537 (2019)
6. Bordes, A., Usunier, N., Chopra, S., Weston, J.: Large-scale simple question answering with memory networks. arXiv preprint arXiv:1506.02075 (2015)
7. Dong, L., Wei, F., Zhou, M., Xu, K.: Question answering over freebase with multi-column convolutional neural networks. In: Proceedings of the 53rd Annual Meeting of the Association for Computational Linguistics and the 7th International Joint Conference on Natural Language Processing (Volume 1: Long Papers) (2015)
8. Hu, S., Zou, L., Yu, J.X., Wang, H., Zhao, D.: Answering natural language questions by subgraph matching over knowledge graphs. IEEE Trans. Knowl. Data Eng. **30**(5), 824–837 (2017)
9. Lan, Y., He, G., Jiang, J., Jiang, J., Zhao, W.X., Wen, J.R.: A survey on complex knowledge base question answering: methods, challenges and solutions. arXiv preprint arXiv:2105.11644 (2021)
10. Min, B., Grishman, R., Wan, L., Wang, C., Gondek, D.: Distant supervision for relation extraction with an incomplete knowledge base. In: Proceedings of the 2013 Conference of the North American Chapter of the Association for Computational Linguistics: Human Language Technologies (2013)
11. Sun, H., Dhingra, B., Zaheer, M., Mazaitis, K., Salakhutdinov, R., Cohen, W.W.: Open domain question answering using early fusion of knowledge bases and text. arXiv preprint arXiv:1809.00782 (2018)

12. Xiong, W., Yu, M., Chang, S., Guo, X., Wang, W.Y.: Improving question answering over incomplete KBS with knowledge-aware reader. arXiv preprint arXiv:1905.07098 (2019)

13. Han, J., Cheng, B., Wang, X.: Open domain question answering based on text enhanced knowledge graph with hyperedge infusion. In: Proceedings of the 2020 Conference on Empirical Methods in Natural Language Processing: Findings (2020)

14. Saxena, A., Tripathi, A., Talukdar, P.: Improving multi-hop question answering over knowledge graphs using knowledge base embeddings. In: Proceedings of the 58th Annual Meeting of the Association for Computational Linguistics (2020)

15. Bordes, A., Usunier, N., Garcia-Duran, A., Weston, J., Yakhnenko, O.: Translating embeddings for modeling multi-relational data. In: Advances in Neural Information Processing Systems, vol. 26 (2013)

16. Nickel, M., Tresp, V., Kriegel, H.P.: A three-way model for collective learning on multi-relational data. In: ICML (2011)

17. Trouillon, T., Welbl, J., Riedel, S., Gaussier, É., Bouchard, G.: Complex embeddings for simple link prediction. In: International Conference on Machine Learning. PMLR (2016)

18. Yih, W.T., Richardson, M., Meek, C., Chang, M.W., Suh, J.: The value of semantic parse labeling for knowledge base question answering. In: Proceedings of the 54th Annual Meeting of the Association for Computational Linguistics (Volume 2: Short Papers (2016)

19. Berant, J., Chou, A., Frostig, R., Liang, P.: Semantic parsing on freebase from question-answer pairs. In: Proceedings of the 2013 Conference on Empirical Methods in Natural Language Processing (2013)

20. Ruffinelli, D., Broscheit, S., Gemulla, R.: You can teach an old dog new tricks! On training knowledge graph embeddings. In: International Conference on Learning Representations (2019)

21. Broscheit, S., Ruffinelli, D., Kochsiek, A., Betz, P., Gemulla, R.: LibKGE-A knowledge graph embedding library for reproducible research. In: Proceedings of the 2020 Conference on Empirical Methods in Natural Language Processing: System Demonstrations (2020)

22. Li, J., et al.: BioCreative V CDR task corpus: a resource for chemical disease relation extraction. Database J. Biol. Databases Curation **2016**, baw068 (2016)

23. Song, Y., Kim, E., Lee, G.G., Yi, B.K.: POSBIOTM-NER in the shared task of BioNLP/NLPBA2004. In: Proceedings of the International Joint Workshop on Natural Language Processing in Biomedicine and its Applications (NLPBA/BioNLP) (2004)

24. Broscheit, S., Ruffinelli, D., Kochsiek, A., Betz, P., Gemulla, R.: LibKGE-A Knowledge Graph Embedding Library for Reproducible Research, pp. 165–174 (2020)

25. Devlin, J., Chang, M., Lee, K., Toutanova, K.: BERT: pre-training of deep bidirectional transformers for language understanding. arXiv preprint arXiv:1810.04805 (2018)

26. Lee, J., et al.: BioBERT: a pre-trained biomedical language representation model for biomedical text mining. Bioinformatics **36**(4), 1234–1240 (2020)

27. Paszke, A., et al.: PyTorch: an imperative style, high-performance deep learning library. In: Advances in Neural Information Processing Systems, vol. 32 (2019)

28. Liu, Y., et al.: Roberta: a robustly optimized BERT pretraining approach. arXiv preprint arXiv:1907.11692 (2019)

29. Wolf, T., et al.: Transformers: State-of-the-Art Natural Language Processing, pp. 38–45 (2020)

30. Kingma, D.P., Ba, J.: Adam: a method for stochastic optimization. arXiv preprint arXiv:1412.6980 (2014)

31. Souza, F., Nogueira, R., Lotufo, R.: Portuguese named entity recognition using BERT-CRF. arXiv preprint arXiv:1909.10649 (2019)

Discovering Combination Patterns of Traditional Chinese Medicine for the Treatment of Gouty Arthritis with Renal Dysfunction

Wenying Chen[1], Weihan Qiu[2], Tao Chen[2], Yiyong Xu[1], Xiaolin Zhang[1],
Xiumin Chen[1,3,4], Runyue Huang[1,3,4], and Maojie Wang[1,3,4(✉)]

[1] The Second Affiliated Hospital of Guangzhou University of Chinese Medicine (Guangdong Provincial Hospital of Chinese Medicine), Guangzhou, China
`{candy011011,ryhuang,maojiewang}@gzucm.edu.cn`
[2] School of Computer Science, South China Normal University, Guangzhou, China
[3] Guangdong Provincial Key Laboratory of Clinical Research on Traditional Chinese Medicine Syndrome, Guangzhou, China
[4] State Key Laboratory of Dampness Syndrome of Chinese Medicine, The Second Affiliated Hospital of Guangzhou University of Chinese Medicine, Guangzhou, China

Abstract. Traditional Chinese Medicine (TCM) can effectively suppress inflammation, reduce serum uric acid levels and improve renal function. However, there is a major challenge to explore effective drug combinations due to the complexity of TCM components and the wide variation in drug prescriptions. Data mining technology provides more accurate drug screening and disease prediction than classical statistical methods. This study explores the usage patterns of TCM for the treatment of gouty arthritis with renal dysfunction for the first time. The original data is the outpatient medical records from the Guangdong Provincial Traditional Chinese Medicine Hospital. The Apriori algorithm and Louvain algorithm are applied to discover how the usages of traditional Chinese medicine are associated and connected. According to the result of Apriori analysis, the Chinese medicine combination *Tufuling* and *Fenbixie* is the most frequently used drug pair for the disease. According to the result of Louvain algorithm, 119 communities are divided and core communities are further extracted. The discoveries are mapped and interpreted for clinical practices.

Keywords: Gouty arthritis with renal dysfunction · Traditional Chinese Medicine · Association rule mining · Louvain algorithm

1 Introduction

Gouty arthritis (gout) is a common inflammatory disease that caused by the deposition of monosodium urate crystals in joints or soft tissues, with a prevalence of 1.1% in China [1] and between 1%–6.8% worldwide [2]. Hyperuricemia is one of the most typical clinical features of gout and is mainly caused by abnormal purine metabolism. Hyperuricemia is also a common trigger for kidney damage. For example, previous

B. Tang et al. (Eds.): CHIP 2022, CCIS 1772, pp. 170–183, 2023.
https://doi.org/10.1007/978-981-19-9865-2_12

studies have shown that the development of hyperuricemia results in kidney damage, accelerating CKD progression and an increase in mortality [3]. The risk of kidney disease has been increased by 7% for each 60 umol/L rise in serum uric acid [4]. Moreover, the long-term administration of NSAIDs and colchicine may result in renal dysfunction and even lead to deterioration of renal function in patients with CKD4 [5]. Therefore, urate-lowering therapy, which works by inhibiting the synthesis of uric acid or promoting its excretion, is the major therapy strategy currently. Existing evidences have shown that effective management and regulation of hyperuricemia contributes significantly to the reduction of gout flares and other relative comorbidities [3, 4]. Unfortunately, the percentage of gout patients achieving 3-month and 6-month serum uric acid regression treatment was only 29.12% and 38.20%, respectively [6].

Renal dysfunction is one of the main comorbidities of gout, and it increases the difficulty of gout treatment. Traditional Chinese Medicine (TCM) is widely practiced in China for the treatment of gouty arthritis. A large amount of clinical evidences have shown that TCM can effectively suppress inflammation, reduce serum uric acid levels and improve renal function under the guidance of TCM evidence-based treatment theory, which indicates that TCM has great potential in the treatment of gouty arthritis with renal dysfunction and is worth exploring and researching. In a large number of prescriptions, the effective drug combinations and core drug communities were summarized, which is beneficial for promoting their application in clinical decision-making and can even be used as the basis for the study of Chinese patent medicines for the treatment of gout. By exploring the core drug communities, it may be possible to get new inspirations or conclusions on the clinical treatment thoughts. However, the complexity of TCM components and the wide variation in drug prescriptions used by practitioners make it a major challenge to explore effective drug combinations. The innovation of this paper is reflected through the connection between gout patients and drug-using-regularity conducted by the Apriori algorithm and Louvain algorithm.

There have been considerable numbers of achievements in data mining technology in the research of TCM, including ones in gout and renal dysfunction fields. Recent technology provides more accurate drug screening and disease prediction for gout and renal function diseases than statistical methods. Li et al. [7] skillfully combined modern pharmacological methods and computer simulation models with traditional medicine, pointing out the direction of TCM in the treatment of diseases in this area. Xia et al. [8] have shown the possibility of exploring TCM treatment strategies using a integrated analysis method. Others also discussed the applications of TCM in gout from different perspectives, such as drug use and statistics on patient treatment [9–11]. The association rule mining algorithm is frequently served as a primary method for data analysis in this field. The Apriori is one of the most widely used methods among the algorithms. The Apriori algorithm aims to generate frequent itemsets with minimum support, and those that meet the threshold of support and confidence are generated afterwards [12]. For the empirical formula, which is important in TCM, the association rule algorithms have played an essential role in sorting out the experience of TCM, as well as finding the relationship among drugs, syndromes, and clinical indexes by analyzing prescriptions [13]. After mining key molecules that affected the properties of cold and heat, combined with the hierarchical clustering algorithm, there were some commonalities in the chemical composition of CHM with the same property [14]. The basic Apriori algorithm could only handle boolean type data, thus Zhang et al. [15] improved the algorithm by incorporating the drug dose into data. This research did not require the conversion of data to Boolean type and also improved the calculation of performance.

Moreover, the purpose of community detection is to explore the community structure hidden behind complex networks to further understand the structure of complex networks. In recent years, complex network-related technologies have been widely used in the field of TCM. Mu et al. [16] extracted the prescriptions for the treatment of systemic lupus erythematosus from the literature, performed complex network analysis, and obtained the core basic prescriptions for the treatment of the disease. Xi et al. [17] used Louvain algorithm to analyze the prescription data with myocardial infarction, and proposed drug regimens for the causes, symptoms and complications of the disease. In order to solve the problem of unstable performance of the label propagation algorithm, Zhang et al. [18] proposed a label propagation algorithm based on label importance. Different from the traditional label propagation algorithm, this algorithm updated node labels in the order of node importance. The algorithm was applied to a drug network to discover drug groups that treat multiple indications.

To that end, this paper proposes to utilize the Apriori algorithm and Louvain algorithm to discover effective usage patterns of TCM. The data was 401 outpatient medical records of 153 patients from Guangdong Provincial Traditional Chinese Medicine Hospital. Exploring the relationship between traditional Chinese medicine for the treatment of gout with renal dysfunction can provide a reference for clinical drug combinations to formulate the best drug regimen and promote the development of new drugs. According to the Apriori analysis, the rules of both uric acid and creatinine decreased with the highest confidence, support and lift values for the patients with renal dysfunction were extracted. According to the community detection, a total of 119 communities was divided and the core communities were extracted, which may serve as a reference for clinical practice.

The main contributions of this paper lies on the three aspects:

1) To the best of our knowledge, this is the first study on exploring the usage patterns of TCM for the treatment of gout with renal dysfunction.
2) Through applying Apriori algorithm in association rule mining and Louvain algorithm for community detection, the effective drug combinations and the core drug communities that lowered uric acid and creatinine as well as for the treatment of gouty arthritis with renal dysfunction were discovered.
3) The experiments present that patients are often associated with poor sleep and throat discomfort, suggesting the necessity of attention to sleep quality and pharynx in the treatment of the disease.

2   The Methodology

2.1   The Overall Workflow

The data is the outpatient medical records diagnosed with gout from the Guangdong Provincial Traditional Chinese Medicine Hospital during 2020–2021, from which the

Chinese medicine prescriptions and the laboratory test index were extracted. Data Masking (hiding the patient's name and medical card number) was performed when the data was obtained from the Information Department, and the acquisition and processing of the data did not violate any ethical principles. Uric acid and creatinine are key indicators of the severity of gouty arthritis with renal dysfunction, so they were used as reference indicators in this study. According to data indexes, the original data were divided into two groups, the urate-lowering group and the creatinine-lowering group. The former was stratified into three subgroups according to the degrees of uric acid decreased (>50%, 20–50%, <20%). Furthermore, a renal dysfunction group with both indexes decreased was extracted.

The overall workflow of this paper is shown in Fig. 1. The data pre-processing mainly aims at transforming the clinical data into a proper format to meet the requirements of algorithms. The raw clinical data are divided into three prescription groups, i.e. the urate-lowering group, the creatinine-lowering group and the abnormal renal function group with both indicators decreased. After that, the analysis of characteristics of TCM are implemented, including indicators of Frequency, Properties, Flavors and Meridian tropism. Our research applies two algorithms: Apriori for associate rule mining and Louvain for community detection.

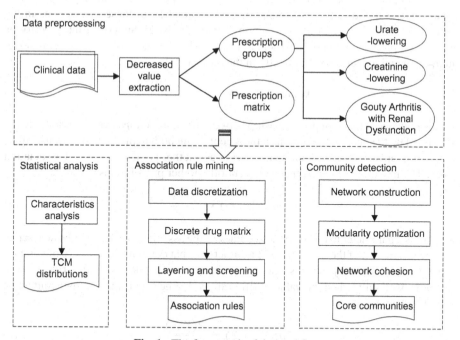

Fig. 1. The framework of the workflow

After the drugs that appeared in the prescription group are collected, the statistics including frequency computation is performed. Then a matrix is generated in the discretization process. The collected drugs are converted to the attributes of the matrix, and the prescription group is as instance. After the discretization of the medicine in the selected prescription group, drugs that appeared in any specific prescription with 1 or 0 are presented as the element of the matrix. The data in the matrix is used for the Apriori analysis.

For Louvain algorithm, drug network is established based on clinical prescriptions for the uric acid decreasing data group. Drugs are replaced by integer numbers. For example, 102 represents *Longgu*. The drugs appearing in the same prescription are connected in pairs. The weight of the edges connected to a drug pair is accumulated. The weighted network is as the input to Louvain algorithm for analysis.

2.2 Apriori Algorithm

Apriori algorithm is one of the association rule mining algorithms in data mining. It identifies the associations and frequent patterns among a set of items in a given database [19, 20]. Formally, an item in the association rule algorithms is a transaction. $X = \{i_1, \ldots, i_m\}$ is defined as a set of transactions. $Y = \{t_1, \ldots, t_n\}$ represents a set of transactions, in which each transaction is a set of items. The itemset refers to any subset of X. The association rule indicates a specific relation between the two itemsets X and Y, where $X \Rightarrow Y$.

The importance of a rule is determined by two parameters, namely support and confidence. Support is the percentage of the combination of these transactions in the dataset. The percentage of all transactions is denoted by T. Support usually performs as the first parameter to build association rules. The threshold of support helps select itemsets which occur more frequently in the dataset.

$$Support(X \Rightarrow Y) = \frac{\sigma(X \cup Y)}{T} \tag{1}$$

Confidence is the strong relationship between the transactions in association rules. It is defined by the percentage of transactions containing both itemsets among transactions containing only itemset X. Confidence serves as another parameter to build association rules. The threshold of confidence helps cut off another pile of itemsets.

$$Confidence(X \Rightarrow Y) = \frac{\sigma(X \cup Y)}{\sigma(X)} \tag{2}$$

Lift is a parameter to evaluate the accuracy of the association rules. It aims at describing the proportion of the probability of transactions that contain Y in the case of containing X to the probability of transactions containing Y only. The association rule $X \Rightarrow Y$ performs well only when the value of lift is above 1. The rule is more convincing when the lift is larger.

$$Lift(X \Rightarrow Y) = \frac{P(Y|X)}{P(Y)} \tag{3}$$

2.3 Louvain Algorithm

Louvain algorithm is a community detection algorithm based on modularity. The modularity Q is a global function proposed by Newman and Girvan for judging the quality of community detection results [21, 22]. Its value range is 0–1. When there are more edges in the community, the larger the Q value, the better the division effect. The calculation is shown in Eq. (4).

$$Q = \frac{1}{2m} \sum_{ij} (A_{ij} - \frac{k_i k_j}{2m}) \times \delta(C_i, C_j) \tag{4}$$

m is the sum of the weights of all edges in network, A_{ij} is the adjacency matrix of the network, k_i and k_j are the sum of all edge weights pointing to node i and node j. $\delta(C_i, C_j)$ indicates whether node i and node j are in the same community. $\delta(C_i, C_j)$ is 1 if both in the same community, otherwise it is 0.

Assuming that the modularity corresponding to the community before the joining of a node is Q, and the modularity corresponding to the community after the movement is Q', and the difference between Q' and Q is the modularity increment ΔQ after the joining. The calculation is shown in Eq. (5).

$$Q = \frac{\sum_{in}}{2m} - \left(\frac{\sum_{tot}}{2m}\right)^2 - \left(\frac{k_i}{2m}\right)^2 \tag{5}$$

$$Q' = \frac{\sum_{in} + k_{i,in}}{2m} - \left(\frac{\sum_{tot} + k_i}{2m}\right)^2 \tag{6}$$

$$\Delta Q = \left[\frac{\sum_{in} + k_{i,in}}{2m} - \left(\frac{\sum_{tot} + k_i}{2m}\right)^2\right] - \left[\frac{\sum_{in}}{2m} - \left(\frac{\sum_{tot}}{2m}\right)^2 - \left(\frac{k_i}{2m}\right)^2\right] \tag{7}$$

$\sum_{in}$ is the weight sum of the edges inside the community, $\sum_{tot}$ is the weight sum of the edges connecting the community to the outside community, k_i is the edge weight sum connected to node i, and $k_{i,in}$ is the edge weight sum connected to node i within the community.

Louvain algorithm is mainly composed of two stages: modularity optimization and network cohesion. At the beginning, each node is regarded as an individual community, and the number of communities is equal to the number of nodes. In the modularity optimization stage, the algorithm traverses the adjacent nodes of each node in the network in turn and add the node into the community where its adjacent nodes belong to. The change value ΔQ of the modularity is calculated and updated after the joining. If ΔQ is a negative value, the node remains in the original community, otherwise it joins the community that maximizes ΔQ. This operation is repeated until the community to which each node of the network belongs does not change. In the network agglomeration stage, the community is condensed into super nodes, the edges between internal nodes of the community are regarded as the ring edges of super nodes, and the edge weights between the super nodes are the sum of the edge weights among communities. The two stages are continuously iterated until the modularity of the entire network reaches the maximum. Each network structure corresponds to a degree of modularity. The degree of modularity corresponding to the network changes when a community changes. Compared with other community detection algorithms, the Louvain algorithm has low complexity, fast convergence speed and good stability, and can be used in large networks.

3 The Results

3.1 Data Analysis

Table 1. Characteristics of the outpatient medical records.

Group	Urate lowering group			Creatinine lowering group	Renal dysfunction group	
	Uric acid decreased >50%	Uric acid decreased 20%–50%	Uric acid decreased <20%	Creatinine decreased	Uric acid decreased	Creatinine decreased
Prescriptions count	14	153	145	216	70	
Average index (before)	679	556.90	387.70	98.02	559.20	112.87
Average index (after)	244	393.67	361.46	90.70	366.30	106.62
Percentage of decreasing	64.06%	29.31%	6.77%	7.47%	34.50%	5.54%

A total of 401 outpatient medical records were divided into three groups including urate-lowering group, creatinine-lowering group and renal dysfunction group according to clinical characteristics. As shown in Table 1, the urate-lowering group was stratified into three subgroups based on the degrees of uric acid decreased (>50%, 20–50%, <20%), with the >50% subgroup containing 14 prescriptions with a 64.06% decreasing in uric acid, the 20–50% subgroup containing 153 prescriptions with 29.31% decreasing and the <20% subgroup containing 145 prescriptions with 6.77% decreasing. There were 216 prescriptions in creatinine-lowering group, which index decreased by 7.47%. A total of 70 prescriptions in the group with renal dysfunction had a 34.50% decreasing in uric acid and a 5.54% decreasing in creatinine.

3.2 Results of Association Rule Mining

In the urate-lowering data group, the drug combinations were obtained by Apriori algorithm. The minimum support was set as 30%, and the minimum confidence was 80%. A total of 36 association rules were extracted and sorted according to the support. The top 10 selected rules discovered from patients whose urate-lowering decreased by more than 50% were presented in Table 2.

Among them, the drug prescriptions with the highest confidence, support and lift values were ranked, where '*Guizhi→Chaoyiyiren*', '*Chaoyiyiren→Guizhi*', '*Cangzhu→Tufuling*'. The drug combinations were *Cangzhu, Guizhi, Tufuling, Chaoyiyiren*, and *Weilingxian*.

Table 2. The top 10 rules extracted from the patients whose urate-lowering decreased by more than 50%.

Rank	Pre-items	Post-items	Support	Confidence	Lift
1	*Guizhi*	*Chaoyiyiren*	50.00	100.00	1.75
2	*Chaoyiyiren*	*Guizhi*	50.00	87.50	1.75
3	*Cangzhu*	*Tufuling*	42.86	85.71	1.50
4	*Fenbixie*	*Cangzhu*	35.71	100.00	2.00
5	*Weilingxian*	*Cangzhu*	35.71	100.00	2.00
6	*Weilingxian*	*Tufuling*	35.71	100.00	1.75
7	*Weilingxian* and *Cangzhu*	*Tufuling*	35.71	100.00	1.75
8	*Weilingxian* and *Tufuling*	*Cangzhu*	35.71	100.00	2.00
9	*Shancigu* and *Guizhi*	*Chaoyiyiren*	35.71	100.00	1.75
10	*Shancigu* and *Chaoyiyiren*	*Guizhi*	35.71	100.00	2.00

In the creatinine-lowering data group, the drug combinations were obtained by Apriori algorithm. The minimum support was set as 13%, and the minimum confidence was 80%. A total of 27 association rules were extracted and sorted according to the support. The top 10 selected rules discovered from patients with creatinine-lowering were presented in Table 3.

Among them, the drug prescriptions with the highest confidence, support and lift values were ranked, where '*Huangbo→Yiyiren*', '*Fenbixie* and *Yiyiren→Tufuling*', '*Huangbo* and *Tufuling→Yiyiren*'. The drug combinations were *Guizhi Zhimu*, *Zexie*, *Tufuling*, *Cangzhu*, *Yiyiren*, *Huangbo*, and *Fenbixie*.

Table 3. The top 10 rules extracted from the patients with creatinine-lowering.

Rank	Pre-items	Post-items	Support	Confidence	Lift
1	*Huangbo*	*Yiyiren*	21.20	90.20	2.08
2	*Fenbixie* and *Yiyiren*	*Tufuling*	18.89	87.23	1.71
3	*Huangbo* and *Tufuling*	*Yiyiren*	16.13	92.11	2.13
4	*Zhimu*	*Zexie*	15.67	80.95	2.22
5	*Fenbixie* and *Cangzhu*	*Tufuling*	15.21	84.62	1.65
6	*Huangbo* and *Cangzhu*	*Yiyiren*	15.21	89.19	2.06
7	*Zelan*	*Baizhu*	15.21	100.00	3.56
8	*Chishao* and *Cangzhu*	*Tufuling*	14.29	83.78	1.64
9	*Zhimu* and *Zexie*	*Guizhi*	12.90	82.35	3.08
10	*Guizhi* and *Zexie*	*Zhimu*	12.90	84.85	4.38

In the renal dysfunction data group, the drug combinations were obtained by Apriori algorithm. The minimum support was set as 20%, and the minimum confidence was 80%. A total of 29 association rules were extracted and sorted according to the support. The top 10 selected rules discovered from patients with both urate-lowering and creatinine-lowering were presented in Table 3.

Among them, the drug prescriptions with the highest confidence, support and lift values were ranked, where '*Fenbixie*→*Tufuling*', '*Yiyiren*→*Tufuling*', '*Yiyiren* and *Fenbixie*→*Tufuling*'. The drug combinations were *Yiyiren, Huangbo, Fenbixie, Tufuling, Cangzhu*, and *Niuxi*.

Table 4. The top 10 rules extracted from the patients with both urate-lowering and creatinine-lowering in renal dysfunction group.

Rank	Pre-items	Post-items	Support	Confidence	Lift
1	*Fenbixie*	*Tufuling*	41.18	82.35	1.33
2	*Yiyiren*	*Tufuling*	38.24	86.67	1.40
3	*Yiyiren* and *Fenbixie*	*Tufuling*	26.47	94.74	1.53
4	*Huangbo*	*Yiyiren*	23.53	94.12	2.13
5	*Cangzhu* and *Niuxi*	*Tufuling*	23.53	84.21	1.36
6	*Cangzhu* and *Tufuling*	*Niuxi*	23.53	80.00	1.75
7	*Weilingxian*	*Tufuling*	22.06	100.00	1.62
8	*Yinchen*	*Fuling*	22.06	88.24	2.50
9	*Chishao*	*Cangzhu*	22.06	88.24	2.31
10	*Huangbo*	*Tufuling*	22.06	88.24	1.43

3.3 Result of Community Detection

By applying Louvain algorithm, drugs as nodes of the same color in the network belonged to the same community. Drugs in the same community were more likely to be prescribed together. The larger the weight of an edge, the darker the color. On the uric acid decreasing dataset, the network was generated and visualized in Fig. 2.

The drug network contained 329 nodes and 6657 edges. The average degree was 40.468, the network diameter was 3, the average path length was 1.827, and the average clustering coefficient was 0.746. A total of 119 communities were identified and the nodes in the same color were extracted to obtain core communities. Combined with clinical treatment experience of gout disease, two core communities, as examples, were displayed in Fig. 3.

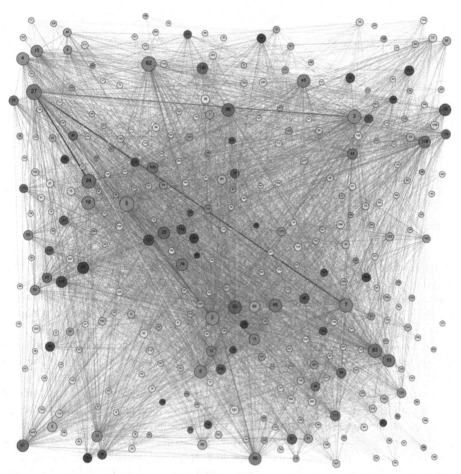

Fig. 2. The generated drug network on the uric acid decreasing data group for gout patients using Louvain algorithm.

4   The Discussion

In the association rule analysis, among the TCM prescriptions that lower uric acid, '*Baizhu*→*Fuling*' is the most frequently used drug pair. In addition, in the prescriptions of potent uric acid-lowering (>50% decreasing after treatment) as shown in Table 2, '*Guizhi*→*Chaoyiyiren*' is most frequently used one. The prescriptions that containing *Baizhu* and *Fuling* such as *Shenling Baizhu Powder* often have a notable therapeutic effect in the treatment of gout [23]. Among them, *Fuling* can lower uric acid through two pathways, one is to promote the excretion of *UA* by regulating intestinal flora [24]. The other is polysaccharides of poria cocos, which is the main component in *Fuling* to increase the excretion of urine uric acid and decrease serum uric acid by up-regulating the expression of OAT1 (organic anion transporter1) and down-regulating the expression of URAT1(urate transporter1) [25]. In this study, the combination of

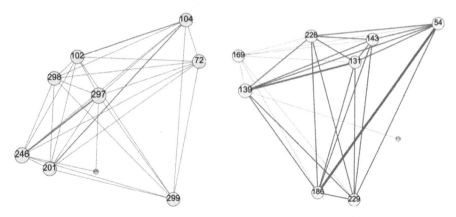

Fig. 3. Two core communities identified from 119 communities using Louvain algorithm.

'*Guizhi*→*Chaoyiyiren*' could reduce uric acid by more than 50%, which may suggest that this combination leads to a more dramatic decrease in uric acid. The main mechanism is that cinnamaldehyde, the main component of *Guizhi* [26], and fat-soluble substances in *Chaoyiyiren* could significantly inhibit xanthine oxidase (XOD) activity, reducing purine catabolism and controlling uric acid levels.

As shown in Table 3, the combination with the highest support and confidence in creatinine-lowering group is '*Huangbo*→*Yiyiren*'. *Huangbo* is used as "principal drug" in the classic formulas *Ermiao San* and *Sanmiao San* for the treatment of gouty arthritis. *Huangbo* can significantly reduce uric acid and creatinine levels and inhibit joint swelling in rats with hyperuricemia [27], while its major ingredient berberine had nephroprotective effects by inhibiting Bax expression, promoting Bcl-2 expression and reducing apoptosis of renal cells [28]. *Yiyiren* extract activates TGF and Toll-like Receptor Signaling Pathways in the kidney, lessening renal interstitial fibrosis and renal tubular epithelial cell apoptosis, thereby reducing the production of inflammatory factors and protecting renal function [29, 30].

As shown in Table 4, the combination '*Fenbixie*→*Tufuling*' had the highest support and confidence in the renal dysfunction group, indicating its efficacy in improving uric acid and creatinine levels. In the TCM perspective, the evil of turbidity and stasis in gouty arthritis with renal dysfunction is more severe and the vital *Qi* is more deficient. *Tufuling* and *Fenbixie* are the "principal drug" and "minister drug" in *Xiezhuo Chubi Decoction*, which work together to drain turbidity and remove blood stasis, strengthen the spleen and remove dampness. In the mechanistic perspective, a network pharmacology study of the "*Tufuling* plus *Fenbixie*" showed that they treated gouty arthritis through the IL-4 signaling pathway, IL-10 signaling pathway, IL-13 signaling pathway, and IL-17 signaling pathway by means of anti-inflammatory immune mechanisms [31]. *Tufuling* both inhibits hepatic XOD activity and reduces purine synthesis [32], and has protective effects against kidney injury [33]. Total saponin of Dioscorea has a regulatory effect on blood uric acid by reducing the reabsorption of uric acid by decreasing the expression of URAT1, as well as promoting uric acid excretion by upregulating the expression of OAT1 and OAT3 (organic anion transporter3) [34].

In the Fig. 3, the core community (left) appears as a group of Chinese medicine with the effect of tranquilizing, which may suggest that patients with gouty arthritis are often associated with poor sleep. A clinical survey in 2018 showed that the prevalence of sleep disorder in patients with gouty arthritis was 55.3% in Chinese [35]. The direct factors that affect sleep are severe pain due to flares and pain due to chronic joint inflammation, as well as indirect factors are comorbidities such as hypertension, sleep apnea or adverse drug reactions [36]. From the perspective of TCM, the disease damages the vital *Qi* over time, resulting in deficiency of essence and blood, and consequently malnutrition of heart and spirit, so the treatment requires nourishing blood for tranquillization. This core community suggests that treatment of the disease should take sleep quality into account.

The core community (right) is a group of clearing heat and relieving sore throat medicine, which may be explained by the phenomena that patients with renal dysfunction are often associated with throat discomfort. Patients with chronic kidney disease often have a history of recurrent tonsillitis, triggering and aggravating kidney disease, which is more apparent in IgA nephropathy, as a survey showed that 64% patients with IgA nephropathy have chronic pharyngitis and tonsillitis [37]. From the perspective of Traditional Chinese medicine, it can be explained by the theory of "pharynx and kidney-related". From the point of view of meridians, the pharynx and the kidney are connected through the meridian, while from the relationship between *zang-fu* viscera, the pharynx and the kidney are in a physiological relationship of gold and water. In addition, it contains the ideology of dispersion and purgation for the treatment of gouty nephropathy via ventilating lung qi for diuresis. This core community suggests the necessity of attention to pharynx in the treatment of gouty arthritis with renal dysfunction.

5 Conclusions

This study explores the usage patterns of traditional Chinese medicine for the treatment of gout with renal dysfunction using associate role mining and community detection algorithms. According to the result of associate role mining, '*Guizhi→Chaoyiyiren*' is the most frequently used drug pair with the highest confidence, support and lift values from patients whose urate-lowering decreased by more than 50%. '*Huangbo→Yiyiren*' is the most frequently used one from patients with creatinine-lowering. '*Fenbixie→Tufuling*' has the highest and support values for the treatment of gouty arthritis with renal dysfunction. According to the result of community detection algorithms, it is necessary to pay attention to sleep quality and pharynx in the treatment of gouty arthritis.

Acknowledgements. This work was supported by the Keypoint Research and Invention Program of Guangdong (2020B1111100010), The China-Dutch special projects of Guangdong Provincial Hospital of Chinese Medicine (YN2019HL02), and The Specific Fund of State Key Laboratory of Dampness Syndrome of Chinese Medicine (SZ2021KF16).

References

1. Liu, R., et al.: Prevalence of Hyperuricemia and gout in Mainland China from 2000 to 2014: a systematic review and meta-analysis. BioMed Res. Int. **2015**, 1–12 (2015)

2. Dehlin, M., Jacobsson, L., Roddy, E.: Global epidemiology of gout: prevalence, incidence, treatment patterns and risk factors. Nat. Rev. Rheumatol. **16**, 380–390 (2020)

3. Giordano, C., Karasik, O., King-Morris, K., Asmar, A.: Uric acid as a marker of kidney disease: review of the current literature. Dis. Mark. **2015**, 1–6 (2015)

4. Tsai, C., Lin, S., Kuo, C., Huang, C.: Serum uric acid and progression of kidney disease: a longitudinal analysis and mini-review. PLOS ONE **12**, e0170393 (2017)

5. Chinese Medical Doctors Association Nephrologist Branch: Chinese practice guideline for the diagnosis and treatment of Hyperuricemia in renal disease (2017 Edition). Nat. Med. J. China, **97** 1927–1936 (2017)

6. Teh, C., Cheong, Y., Wan, S., Ling, G.: Treat-to-target (T2T) of serum urate (SUA) in gout: a clinical audit in real-world gout patients. Reumatismo **71**, 154–159 (2019)

7. Li, X., Wang, H.: Chinese herbal medicine in the treatment of chronic kidney disease. Adv. Chronic Kidney Dis. **12**, 276–281 (2005)

8. Xia, P., et al.: Data mining-based analysis of Chinese medicinal herb formulae in chronic kidney disease treatment. Evid. Based Complement. Altern. Med. **2020**, 1–14 (2020)

9. Wang, Y., et al.: Optimized project of traditional Chinese medicine in treating chronic kidney disease stage 3: a multicenter double-blinded randomized controlled trial. J. Ethnopharmacol. **139**, 757–764 (2012)

10. Yin, R., et al.: The rate of adherence to urate-lowering therapy and associated factors in Chinese gout patients: a cross-sectional study. Rheumatol. Int. **37**(7), 1187–1194 (2017). https://doi.org/10.1007/s00296-017-3746-x

11. Chen, Y., et al.: The prevalence of gout in mainland China from 2000 to 2016: a systematic review and meta-analysis. J. Public Health **25**(5), 521–529 (2017). https://doi.org/10.1007/s10389-017-0812-5

12. Chen, T., Luo, M., Fu, H., Chen, D., Hu, Q., Deng, N.: Application of NER and association rules to traditional Chinese medicine patent mining. In: 2020 International Conferences on Internet of Things (iThings) and IEEE Green Computing and Communications (Green-Com) and IEEE Cyber, Physical and Social Computing (CPSCom) and IEEE Smart Data (SmartData) and IEEE Congress on Cybermatics (Cybermatics) (2020)

13. Li, H., Jiamin, Y., Zhimin, Y., Huanyu, L., Chunhua, H.: Research on the drugs of addition and subtraction of empirical formula of traditional Chinese medicine based on association rules. In: 2013 IEEE International Conference on Bioinformatics and Biomedicine (2013)

14. Xie, F., Wang, L., Zhang, S., Zhang, L., Wang, X.: Research on key molecules of cold and hot properties Chinese herbal medicine based on improved atomic association rules algorithm and hierarchical clustering algorithm. In: Proceedings of the 3rd International Conference on Data Science and Information Technology (2020)

15. Yadong, Z., Kongfa, H., Tao, Y.: Mining effect of famous Chinese medicine doctors on lung-cancer based on association rules. In: 2019 IEEE International Conference on Bioinformatics and Biomedicine (BIBM) (2019)

16. Mu, Y., et al.: Based on the network analysis of traditional Chinese medicine for the treatment of systemic lupus erythematosus disease medication rules. China J. Integr. Tradit. Chin. West. Med. **41**, 199–203 (2021)

17. Xi, J., Wei, R., Xie, Y., Liu, F., Sun, C., Hou, H.: Research on the real-world superiority scheme of Shengmai injection in the treatment of myocardial infarction based on Louvain algorithm. Pharmacol. Clin. Med. Tradit. Chin. Med. **38**, 131–136 (2022)

18. Zhang, Y., Liu, Y., Li, Q., Jin, R., Wen, C.: LILPA: a label importance based label propagation algorithm for community detection with application to core drug discovery. Neurocomputing **413**,107–133 (2020)

19. Yuan, X.: An improved Apriori algorithm for mining association rules. In: AIP Conference Proceedings (2017)

20. Zulfikar, W., Wahana, A., Uriawan, W., Lukman, N.: Implementation of association rules with apriori algorithm for increasing the quality of promotion. In: 2016 4th International Conference on Cyber and IT Service Management (2016)

21. Girvan, M., Newman, M.: Community structure in social and biological networks. In: Proceedings of the National Academy of Sciences, pp. 7821–7826 (2002)

22. Newman, M., Girvan, M.: Finding and evaluating community structure in networks. Phys. Rev. E. **69**(2), 026113 (2004)

23. Liu, L., Qin, L., Shao, F., Yang, X., Long, X., Cai, H.: Effects of modified Shenling Baizhu powder on efficacy and prognosis of gouty arthritis. Liaoning J. Tradit. Chin. Med. **49**, 91–94 (2022)

24. Wang, K., Wu, S., Li, P., Xiao, N., Du, B.: Effects of Poria Cocos on renal injury and gut microbiota in Hyperuricemia rats. Food Sci. **43**, 1–13 (2022)

25. Deng, M., Yan, J., Wang, P., Zhou, Y., Wu, X.: Effects of Pachman on the expression of renal tubular transporters rURAT1, rOAT1 and rOCT2 of the rats with Hyperuricemia. W. J. Tradit. Chin. Med. **32**, 10–14 (2019)

26. Lee, Y., Son, E., Kim, S., Lee, Y., Kim, O., Kim, D.: Synergistic uric acid-lowering effects of the combination of chrysanthemum indicum Linne flower and Cinnamomum cassia (L.) J. Persl Bark extracts. Evid.-Based Complement. Altern. Med. **2017**, 1–9 (2017)

27. Lian, L., Jia, T.: Effects of CORTEX PHELLODENDRI and its processed products on antigout. J. Anhui Agri. **39**, 8911–8912 (2011)

28. Zheng, H., Lan, J., Li, J., Lv, L.: Therapeutic effect of berberine on renal ischemia-reperfusion injury in rats and its effect on Bax and Bcl-2. Exp. Ther. Med. **16**, 2008–2012 (2018)

29. Peng, X., Chen, L., Xue, L.: Effect and mechanism of Coix seed extract on renal function in diabetic nephropathy rats. China J. Mod. Med. **32**, 10–15 (2022)

30. Zhao, M., et al.: In Vitro and In Vivo studies on Adlay-derived seed extracts: phenolic profiles, antioxidant activities, serum uric acid suppression, and xanthine oxidase inhibitory effects. J. Agric. Food Chem. **62**, 7771–7778 (2014)

31. Bai, Z., et al.: A network pharmacology approach to explore the functional mechanisms of Bixie and Tufuling for treating gouty arthritis. J. Hainan Med. Univ. **2016**, 611–617 (2020)

32. Liang, G., et al.: Protective effects of Rhizoma smilacis glabrae extracts on potassium oxonate- and monosodium urate-induced hyperuricemia and gout in mice. Phytomedicine **59**, 152772 (2019)

33. Liu, C., Kang, Y., Zhou, X., Yang, Z., Gu, J., Han, C.: Rhizoma smilacis glabrae protects rats with gentamicin-induced kidney injury from oxidative stress-induced apoptosis by inhibiting caspase-3 activation. J. Ethnopharmacol. **198**, 122–130 (2017)

34. Chen, G., Zhu, L., Na, S., Li, L.: Effect of total saponin of Dioscorea on chronic hyperuricemia and expression of URAT1 in rats. Zhongguo Zhong yao za zhi = Zhongguo zhongyao zazhi = China Journal of Chinese materia medica **38**, 2348–2353 (2013)

35. Fu, T., et al.: AB0898 sleep quality is associated with alcohol use and functional capacity in Chinese patients with gout: a cross-sectional study. Abstracts Accepted for Publication (2017)

36. Singh, J.: Any sleep is a dream far away: a nominal group study assessing how gout affects sleep. Rheumatology **57**, 1925–1932 (2018)

37. Mestecky, J., Novak, J., Moldoveanu, Z., Raska, M.: IgA nephropathy enigma. Clin. Immunol. **172**, 72–77 (2016)

Automatic Classification of Nursing Adverse Events Using a Hybrid Neural Network Model

Xiaowei Ge[1], Kaixia Li[2], Juan Ding[3], Fei Li[4], and Ming Cheng[1(✉)]

[1] Medical Information Department, The First Affiliated Hospital of Zhengzhou University, Zhengzhou, China
fccchengm@zzu.edu.cn
[2] Nursing Department, The First Affiliated Hospital of Zhengzhou University, Zhengzhou, China
[3] Medical Quality Control Department, The First Affiliated Hospital of Zhengzhou University, Zhengzhou, China
[4] School of Cyber Science and Engineering, Wuhan University, Wuhan, China

Abstract. Nursing adverse event means an abnormal event in the process of nursing that causes or may cause adverse outcomes to patients and their families. Its ability to damage personal health or increase the economic burden of patients. At present, the analysis of nursing adverse event report mainly focuses on its structured report content. However, the unstructured text content in the report contains the whole process of the event, but it is often ignored. To tackle this problem, this study proposed a hybrid neural network model for adverse nursing event reports. It uses convolutional neural network and attention based short-term memory to extract text features respectively, and combines structured data. Finally, a feature fusion mechanism is proposed to fuse features at the same scale. To evaluate the proposed method, we constructed a private data set which contained 13265 reports of Chinese nursing adverse events, and compared our method with other currently popular methods. Experimental results show that the proposed model achieves 84.4% f-measure in this task. The comparison results of different models prove that our model is superior to the traditional statistical model, and has better effectiveness and applicability.

Keywords: Hybrid neural network · Chinese nursing adverse events · Classification of event · Deep learning

1 Introduction

With the rapid development of information technology and the continuous updating of hospital information systems, the current nursing data show an explosive growth [1,2]. Especially in recent years, the quality and safety of clinical medical has received more and more attention. Medical adverse events have

© The Author(s), under exclusive license to Springer Nature Singapore Pte Ltd. 2023
B. Tang et al. (Eds.): CHIP 2022, CCIS 1772, pp. 184–196, 2023.
https://doi.org/10.1007/978-981-19-9865-2_13

a high incidence, great impact and serious consequences. It not only affects patient's diagnosis results, increases the patient's pain and economic burden, but it could also cause medical disputes or medical accidents. Because nurses have long contact with patients and low fault tolerance rate [3–5]. The number of nursing adverse events have approached half of all medical adverse events [6]. Nowadays, an electronic nursing adverse event reporting system has been introduced in most hospitals in China. It has record a large number of nursing adverse events reports. However, The level of nursing adverse events is usually determined by the individual, which may lead to deliberate reduction of events level due to human factors [7,8]. Nursing adverse event reports contain a large number of structured and unstructured data, among which unstructured text data describes the whole process of the event. However, in the reporting stage, the content of nursing adverse event reporting is not standardized and cannot be unified and institutionalized. The reporting standards of various medical institutions are not uniform which result in unstructured reported content such as narration and description of the process of the event. Moreover, these procedures lack reasonable classification features and problems such as difficult manual analysis and many human factors [9].

Recently, the deep learning method has achieved the most advanced performance in natural language processing tasks [10,11].However, many tasks are only for unstructured text data, with less assistance from structured data. Due to the limitation of data privacy protection, there are few applications in the field of nursing documents. Lu et al. [12]used deep learning methods to deal with text data of nursing adverse events, but the methods are more traditional. In addition, some researchers propose to combine them through feature fusion, and add the features of structured data to the model.

Inspired by these researchers, For the classification of nursing adverse event reports, we constructed a private data set which contained 13265 reports of Chinese nursing adverse events, and proposed a hybrid neural network model. It uses convolutional neural network and attention based short-term memory to extract text features respectively, and combines structured data to introduce a feature fusion mechanism. Finally, our method is compared with other popular methods.

The main contributions of this article are as follows:

(1) We constructed a data set containing a large complete reports of nursing adverse events in China, which includes four levels of nursing adverse events according to the severity of the events.
(2) We propose a hybrid neural network model, which uses convolutional neural network and attention based short-term memory to extract text features respectively, and combines structured data to propose a feature fusion mechanism.
(3) Conduct extensive and large-scale empirical research to assess the effectiveness of our approach.

2   Related Work

The analysis and processing of clinical information is of great significance to the management of medical quality and safety. In order to intelligently and effectively analyze the report of nursing adverse events, Cao et al. [13] developed and implemented the hospital nursing adverse event reporting system, but the analysis of nursing adverse events in the system is mainly for structured data. Clark et al. [14] used Bayesian algorithm to analyze the correlation with the same adverse events in clinical trials of a large number of approved drugs. Tomita et al. [15] used TextMiningStudio to analyze adverse events related to medical text data such as electronic health records in nursing services. Roy et al. [16] proposed a machine learning model to improve the technology used to assess and predict the risk of adverse events associated with a variety of chronic diseases. Dev et al. [17] automatically classified adverse events in drug vigilance through traditional machine learning.

According to the above, at present, the research on nursing adverse events still lies in the statistics and analysis of structured data. Its unstructured text information describes the cause, process and result of nursing adverse events, which is very important. However, the research on unstructured text information in nursing adverse events is still relatively few. Pooja [18] et al. proposed a least squares double support vector machine (LS-TWSVM) method for text segmentation. Zhuo et al. [19] proposed a KNN based news text classification method. Although these methods improve the effect of text classification to a certain extent, they all need to manually extract text features, and do not consider the correlation between features.

With the deepening of research, convolution neural network (CNN) is one of the most popular deep learning algorithms in recent years. Kim [20]designed a TEXTCNN model, which is simple and efficient in text classification. GAO YL et al. [21] proposed an improved CNN short text classification model, which can extract short text features of different granularity, and has a high classification accuracy. Song et al. [22] analyzed the feasibility of Chinese nursing adverse event text by verifying natural language processing. Yin et al. [23] found that CNN has shorter training time and better text classification effect than RNN in text classification through comparative experiments.

Although CNN and its improved model can effectively extract local key information, it ignores text context semantic information.Long Short Term Memory (LSTM), a variant of recurrent neural network (RNN), can extract contextual semantic information of text and mine local features of data. CNN and LSTM have their own advantages in extracting text information. But their interpretability is relatively weak. To this end, Bahdanau et al. [24] introduced the Attention mechanism into RNN and achieved good results in machine translation tasks. Li et al. [25] proposed a dual channel attention model (DCAM) for text emotion analysis. It uses CNN and LSTM for feature extraction, and introduces attention mechanism to focus on important words, which improves the prediction effect of the model. Cheng et al. [26] used hybrid neural networks to predict the outcome of blood culture items with significant results.

Therefore, in order to make full use of the effective information in the unstructured text and unstructured content of nursing adverse events. In the present study, we used the hybrid neural network method to evaluate the constructed real data set.

Information on reporting of nursing adverse events

上报人(Submitted by)：***   日期(Date)：2019-12-26   患者姓名(Patient's name)：***

Structured Indicators

科室(Department Code)：心血管内科 1714(Cardiovascular Medicine 1714)

性别（Sex）:女 2(Female 2)   发生时间(Time of occurrence)：下午 2(Afternoon 2)

护理层级(Levels of care)：2   学历(Education)：大学本科 2(Undergraduate 2)

职称(Job Title)：护师 3(Nurse Practitioner 3)   工作年限(Years of work)：7

患者年龄(Patient's age)：67

患者诊断编码(Patient diagnosis code)：房颤射频消融后 I97.907(After radiofrequency ablation of atrial fibrillation I97.907)

事件类别(Event Category)：药物类(Drugs)

Textual description

护士给 1 床患者输液配置丹参组液体时，误将 4IU 正规胰岛素配置为 41IU 正规胰岛素，于 17:05 为患者输注，18：00 患者诉心慌，大汗淋漓，立即告知值班医师，遵医嘱予吸氧 3L/min、BP:179/103mmHg、p:125 次/分，心电监护示波：房颤；立即建立静脉通路，协助患者平卧位休息，...

（At 17:00, the nurse mistakenly configured 4 IU of regular insulin as 41 IU of regular insulin during the infusion configuration of salvia group fluid, and gave the infusion to the patient in bed 1 at 17:05. At 18:00, the patient complained of panic and profuse sweating, and the nurse immediately informed the physician on duty and gave 3L/min of oxygen as ordered, BP: 179/103 mmHg, p: 125 beats/min, and ECG monitor showed waves: atrial fibrillation. Establish intravenous access immediately and assist the patient to rest in a flat position....）

Fig. 1. Nursing adverse event reporting information

3 Methods

3.1 Task Modeling

As shown in Fig. 1, nursing adverse event reports usually include two parts: structured indicators (event occurrence time, party name, nursing level, patient information, self-evaluation event level, etc.) and text information (describing the whole process of the event). Among them, the event level of self-assessment generally needs to be reviewed and determined by nursing quality experts, this task aims to construct a model to automatically classify nursing adverse events according to their severity. We model the task based on the following steps.

- We construct a dataset D from the real original nursing adverse event reporting content, where the n-level nursing adverse events are denoted as $D_n \in D$.
- In the training phase, we use a dataset D containing D_n, $n \in \{0, 1, 2\}$ to train the model M.
- In the testing phase, we use the already trained model M to predict the level of occurrence of nursing adverse events, thus achieving automatic classification of the level.

3.2   Hybrid Network Model

Our proposed hybrid neural network model including three main parts: Attention based LSTM, CNN and Autoencoder, the whole architecture of our method can be found in Fig. 2. Text information is a description of the whole process of nursing adverse events. There is a lot of useful information in it, and it is important to analyze the events. In addition, the automatic encoder is used to learn the continuous representation of structured indicators in event reports.

Text Representation of Events. Due to the great difference between Chinese and English texts, there is no separator between words. At present, there is no Chinese word segmentation tool, specifically for medicine, nursing and other fields. Google's open-source BERT model [27,28] uses a large number of text corpora and superior computing resources to obtain a Chinese based pre-training language model. This solves the problem of polysemy caused by Word2vec [29], and better represents the semantic information at the sentence level. Therefore, in this study, BERT is selected as the way of text vectorization, which can represent the features of text in Chinese nursing adverse events as deeply as possible.

First, we use BERT pre-trained language model to encode words and get corresponding word vectors. Then, CNN is used to convolve and pool the text matrix to extract the local key features. At the same time, LSTM is used to extract the context features of the text, and the output of LSTM is used as the input of the Attention layer to extract the Attention score [30]. According to the score, the vector of the text passing through the attention layer is calculated. Finally, two output vectors of LSTM-Attention and CNN are obtained.

(1) Input a preprocessed text data set T, where $T = \{t1, t2, ..., tn\}$. The pre-trained BERT model was used to convert each word in T into a vector of fixed length, the word vector is obtained with sentence encoding and position encoding. They are input together as features into BERT's bidirectional Transformer, and finally, the word vector sequence S is obtained, $S = \{s1, s2, ..., sn\}$, where sn is the output vector representation of the sth text.

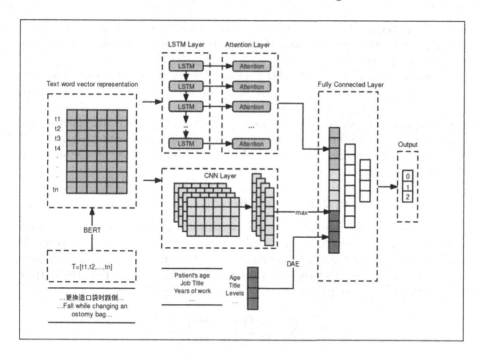

Fig. 2. Hybrid neural network model

(2) CNN consists of several convolution layers, Pooling layers and full connection layers. The convolution layer extracts features through convolution kernels of different sizes. Pooling layer compresses the input feature map to simplify the computational complexity and extract the main features. The full connection layer connects all features and sends the output value to the classifier. First, the text is represented as a matrix, and then the word vectors are convoluted using several convolution cores of different sizes. Maximum pooling of convoluted results yields a new eigenvector $F1$.

(3) LSTM adds input gate i, amnesia gate f, output gate o, and internal memory units to the neurons, which makes it more advantageous in dealing with long sequences of text. It can alleviate the phenomenon of gradient disappearance and explosion, and extract text context information more effectively than RNN. When the input text word vector matrix $S = \{s1, s2, ..., sn\}$, then the update formula of LSTM.

$$i_t = \sigma \left(W_i \cdot [H_{t-1}, s_t] + b_i \right) \tag{1}$$

$$o_t = \sigma \left(W_o \cdot [H_{t-1}, s_t] + b_o \right) \tag{2}$$

$$f_t = \sigma \left(W_f \cdot [H_{t-1}, s_t] + b_f \right) \tag{3}$$

$$C_t = f_t \otimes C_{t-1} + i_t \otimes \tanh \left(W_c \cdot [H_{t-1}, s_t] + b_c \right) \tag{4}$$

$$H_t = o_t \otimes \tanh \left(C_t \right) \tag{5}$$

where H_t is the final output, $\sigma(\cdot)$ is the Sigmoid activation function, $tanh(\cdot)$ is the hyperbolic tangent function, W is the corresponding weight, and b is the corresponding bias value.

Attention mechanism is the distribution of a set of weight values. The word with the largest weight is also the most important in the whole text and plays a greater role in the whole classification task. Therefore, focusing on words that have a greater impact on text results can effectively improve the effect of text classification.We use the output of text context information extracted by LSTM as input to the Attention layer and calculate the match score of the output to the entire eigenvector at each time.

$$score\left(\bar{H}, H_t\right) = W^T rReLU\left(W\bar{H} + UH_t + b\right) \qquad (6)$$

where $\bar{H}$ is a higher level of text representation than the word vector, which is initialized and updated as the model is trained. The higher the score, the more attention, and the most important word. Calculate the overall percentage of output score at each moment, $j \in [0, L]$, Then sum and average the outputs at all times to get the final vector $F2$.

$$F2 = \sum_{i=0}^{L} \frac{\exp\left(score\left(\bar{H}, H_t\right)\right)}{\sum_j score\left(\bar{H}, H_t\right)} H_i \qquad (7)$$

Numerical Representation of Events. Structured indicators in nursing adverse event reports are also of great significance in the analysis and research of nursing adverse events. In this task, the vector dimension of structured data is much smaller than that of embedded text data. In order to avoid the structured data being flooded by high-dimensional text data, we use a denoising automatic encoder (DAE) to amplify the structured data. Set the number of hidden layer nodes to be greater than the input layer to add data dimensions. First, the Dropout layer randomly loses part of the original data x to get $\hat{x}$, Then input it to the encoder to get a hidden vector representation y. The decoder $g(y)$ maps the hidden layer data back to the reconstruction z by reconstructing the low dimension code, and finally gets $F3$

$$\hat{x} = dropout(x) \qquad (8)$$

$$y = f(\hat{x}) = S_f\left(W\hat{x} + b_y\right) \qquad (9)$$

$$z = g(y) = S_g\left(W'y + b_z\right) \qquad (10)$$

where W, b_y are the weight and bias matrix of the encoder, S_f is the nonlinear activation function, W', b_z are the parameters of the decoder, and S_g is the activation function of the decoder.

Feature Fusion and Output Layer. We get the feature vector F1 of CNN after maximum pooling, the output vector F2 of Attention based LSTM, and the vector F3 of structured data after amplification. Three vectors are spliced to get a new vector, and the vector is compressed through three full connection layers. Finally, SVM multi classifier is used to classify them.

4 Experiments

4.1 Data Set Structure and Data Pre-processing

In order to build the data set of this task, we collected a large number of real data reported by nursing adverse events. These data are from the nursing adverse event system of the First Affiliated Hospital of Zhengzhou University, which includes 13911 reported nursing adverse events from March 2014 to December 2019. The data set includes different scenarios such as operation, pipeline, skin, blood transfusion, medicine, falling into bed, etc.

The group standard "Medical Safety (Adverse) Event Management (2018)" issued by China Hospital Association [31]. This standard describes the management specifications of medical institutions in terms of medical safety (adverse) events, including event management, event prevention and control, continuous improvement, etc. This standard is divided into four levels for adverse events: Level I Event (Warning Event), unexpected death or permanent loss of function caused by non natural progression of disease; Level II Event (Error Event): damage to the body and function caused by diagnosis and treatment activities rather than the disease itself in the medical process; Level III Event (Critical Error), although an error has occurred, it has not caused any damage to the body or function, or has minor consequences and can be fully recovered without any treatment; Level IV Event (Near Miss): an event that, due to timely discovery, errors were found and corrected before implementation, and did not cause harm.

In this study, a expert team (composed of multiple experts in nursing management, medical quality control, etc. as well as several nurses) was set up, with 80% of the members having worked in related clinical settings for more than six years. Data inclusion and exclusion criteria were developed. There were no fewer than 600 samples of individual levels of care adverse events. Descriptive content of care adverse events in the report was not empty. Delete reports with missing content, duplicate reports, and descriptions of serious logic errors. The expert team shall refer to the standards and rules, remove some incomplete data, review the event level in the report, and make amendments after negotiation according to experience. Finally, correct data will be formed for the experiment.

After data preprocessing, 646 cases of missing, duplicated, invalid data were excluded. Finally, 13265 cases of data were included, and the effective rate of data was 95.36%. Among them, Level I Events accounted for about 0.6%, Level II Events accounted for about 14.4%, Level III Events accounted for about 52%, and Level IV Events accounted for about 32%. Because of the small amount of Level I Event data, the Level I and Level II Events were combined and analyzed during the study. The data set distribution is shown in Table 1.

Table 1. Data set level classification.

Event Level	Size
Class I events (warning events) AND Class II events (error events)	2069
Class III events (critical errors)	6901
Class IV event (attempted event)	4295

4.2   Evaluation Metrics

In this paper, we chose precision (Pre), recall (Rec), and F-measure to evaluate the effectiveness of classifying the level of occurrence of nursing adverse events.

$$Pre = \frac{TP}{TP + FP} \tag{11}$$

$$Rec = \frac{TP}{TP + FN} \tag{12}$$

$$F - measure = \frac{2 * Pre * Rec}{Pre + Rec} \tag{13}$$

where TP is the grouping of identical adverse events into one category, FP is the grouping of dissimilar adverse nursing events into one category, and similarly, Rec is calculated based on the grouping of dissimilar adverse nursing events into different categories and the grouping of identical ones into different categories.

4.3   Experimental Settings

We follow a ten-fold cross-validation approach, where the entire dataset is divided into ten parts, hich is decoded by the model trained in the remaining parts. We randomly select one of nine training sections as the validation dataset, and for each training procedure performed on the training set, the performance of the model needs to be evaluated once on the validation set. Based on the state of the network model performance on the validation set, the method is simple and effective, and the short training time often produces good results in experiments. In this experiments,To prevent fitting in CNN, Attention-based LSTM network layer. Set drop out value is 0.5, and 50% of the hidden layer units are randomly inactivated. The Relu activation function is used to accelerate the convergence rate and further prevent the occurrence of over-fitting. Set the loss function to be the cross-entropy loss commonly used in multi-classification tasks. The optimizer is Adam, Epoch is 10, Batch size is 256, and the specific parameters are shown in Table 2.

5   Results

In this section, we evaluate the performance of our hybrid model by its ability to accurately predict the level of occurrence of nursing adverse events. We designed multiple sets of experiments for comparison.

Table 2. Parameter settings of the model

Parameter Name	Value	Parameter Name	Value
Word vector dimension	200	CNN convolutional kernel size	2,3,4
Learning rate	0.001	Epochs	10
Hidden layer size	256	Batch size	256
drop out	0.5	Activation function	ReLu

First, we compare the traditional text vectorization methods based on TF-IDF (Term frequency-inverse document frequency) and use different classifiers for Chinese classification. After using the Chinese word segmentation module in Jieba to partition the text and delete the stop words, TF-IDF is used to achieve text vectorization and other pre-processing operations. Logistic regression, random forest, SVM and other classifiers are used to classify the forest. Table 3 shows the results of the classification.

Table 3. Effect of Chinese text classification model based on TF-IDF (%)

Model	Precision	Recall	F-measure
TF-IDF - LogisticRegression	69.21	66.55	67.85
TF-IDF - RandomForest	69.36	62.02	65.48
TF-IDF - SVM	68.16	66.41	67.27

We know that the classification of SVM is better based on TF-IDF model, but the precision of these three methods is below 70% with F-measure, which is generally not good. This may be related to the feature hierarchy of TF-IDF extracting text and the feature of unstructured text in event reports.

Then, we use char-CNN to extract text features of Chinese nursing adverse events, and classify event levels according to CNN's own softmax classifier or 1-to-1 SVM classifier. The results are shown in Table 4.

Table 4. Effect of Chinese text classification model based on The character-level CNN-SVM (%)

Model	Precision	Recall	F-measure
CNN - softmax	70.01	70.34	70.17
CNN - SVM	78.21	75.64	76.90

Chinese nursing adverse events classification model based on character level CNN and classified by softmax or SVM, and traditional classification model based on TF-IDF feature extraction method. F-measure and precision on test sets are better than the two models. The precision of the character-level CNN-SVM classification model is the highest, with an average precision of 78%. The reason may be that CNN convolution neural network can extract deeper features from Chinese nursing adverse events text. However, the structured content of the report on adverse nursing events was not considered.

Based on the structured data and unstructured text content in the report, the model presented in this study can be seen in Table 5. By integrating CNN, Attention-based LSTM, DAE, etc., 84.4% of the F-measures in the classification of adverse nursing event reports could be achieved, which was significantly higher than other methods. It is worth noting that a combination of structured metrics and event text yields better results than text-only features. This is because different types of metrics in structured data can contribute. Only the text description of the reported event is used as input, and the structured information on the adverse event report is ignored, which limits the performance of the task. Additionally, the Attention mechanism was introduced to calculate the Attention Score, which could focus attention on the key words in the structured text of the nursing adverse events report.

Table 5. Effect of Chinese text classification model based on Hybrid Neural Network model (%)

Model	Precision	Recall	F-measures
CNN+LSTM	82.12	80.06	81.08
CNN+LSTM+Attention	84.09	84.81	84.45
CNN+LSTM+Attention+DAE	84.37	84.38	84.38

6   Conclusion

This paper constructed a data set containing a large complete reports of nursing adverse events in China and propose a hybrid neural network for classification of nursing adverse event reports. It uses convolutional neural network and attention based short-term memory to extract text features respectively, and combines structured data to propose feature fusion mechanism. This model can effectively classify nursing adverse event reports and assist in the analysis of adverse events. In our future work, we intend to continue to integrate pre-care adverse events. Further develop an intelligent early warning system for nursing adverse events to assist clinical nurses in making decisions.

Acknowledgments. This work was supported by the Key Project of Science and Technology Research of Henan Province (No. 222102210112), the National Natural and Science Fund of China (No. 61802350, 81971615), National Key Research and Development Program of China (No. 2019YFC0118803).

References

1. O'Brien, R.L., O'Brien, M.W.: Nursing Orientation to Data Science and Machine Learning. Am. J. Nurs. Official Mag. Am. Nurses' Assoc. **121**(4), 32–39 (2021)
2. Drayton-Brooks, S.M., Gray, P.A., Turner, N.P., Newland, J.A.: The use of big data and data mining in nurse practitioner clinical education. J. Prof. Nurs. **36**(6), 484–489 (2020)
3. Liu, Y., Liu, H.P.: Establishing nursing adverse events' reporting content of hospital: using the Delphi method: Frontiers of. Nurs. **7**(4), 337–344 (2020)
4. Choi, S., Cho, E., Kim, E., Lee, K., Chang, S. J.: Effects of nurse staffing, work environment, education on adverse events in nursing homes. Sci. Rep. **11**, 21458 (2021)
5. An, S.L., Wang, L.: Analysis and application of nursing adverse event data based on hospital information platform. Chin. Nurs. Manage. **18**(9), 1153–1156 (2019)
6. Duarte, S.C.M., Stipp, M.A.C., Silva, M.M.: Adverse events and safety in nursing care. Revista brasileira de enfermagem **68**, 144–154 (2015)
7. Yang, X., Wang, X., Shao, W.L.: Analysis of the nursing adverse events based on 335 cases from the reporting system. Chin. J. Nurs. **45**(2), 130–132 (2010)
8. Min, J.K., Jang, S.G., Kim, I.S., Lee, W.: A study on the status and contributory factors of adverse events due to negligence in nursing care. J. Patient Safety **17**(8), e904–e910 (2021)
9. Zang, X., Bai, J.J.: Application of information technology in the management of adverse care events. Chin. J. Nurs. Educ. **14**(1), 29–33 (2017)
10. Alawad, M., Yoon, H.J., Gao, S., Mumphrey, B., Tourassi, G.: Privacy-preserving deep learning NLP models for cancer registries. IEEE Trans. Emerg. Top. Comput. **PP**(99), 1 (2020)
11. Cheng, M., Ge, X.W., Li, K.X.: Research on text classification of adverse nursing events based on CNN-SVM. Comput. Eng. Sci. **42**(1), 161–166 (2020)
12. Lu, W., Jiang, W., Zhang, N., Xue, F.: A deep learning-based text classification of adverse nursing events. J. Healthcare Eng. **2021**, 2094–2107 (2021)
13. Cao, Y., Ball, M.: A hospital nursing adverse events reporting system project: an approach based on the systems development life cycle. Stud. Health Technol. Inform. **245**, 1351 (2017)
14. Clark, M.: Prediction of clinical risks by analysis of pre-clinical and clinical adverse events. J. Biomed. Inform. **54**(C), 167–173 (2015)
15. Tomita, M., Kishi, N., Iwasawa, M.: The analysis of medical adverse events related to electronic health records in nursing services. Studies in Health Technol. Inform. **245**, 1340 (2017)
16. Roy, S.B., Maria, M., Wang, T., Ehlers, A., Flum, D.: Predicting adverse events after surgery. Big Data Res. **13**, 29–37 (2018)
17. Dev, S., Zhang, S., Voyles, J., Rao, A.S.: Automated classification of adverse events in pharmacovigilance. In: 2017 IEEE International Conference on Bioinformatics and Biomedicine (BIBM), pp. 905–909(2017)
18. Saigal, P., Khanna, V.: Multi-category news classification using support vector machine based classifiers. SN Appl. Sci. **2**(3), 1–12 (2020). https://doi.org/10.1007/s42452-020-2266-6
19. Chen, Z., Zhou, L.J., Li, X.D., Zhang, J.N., Huo, W.J.: The lao text classification method based on KNN - ScienceDirect.: Procedia Comput. Sci. **166**, 523–528 (2020)

20. Kim, Y.: Convolutional neural networks for sentence classification. In: Proceedings of the 2014 Conference on Empirical Methods in Natural Language Processing (EMNLP), pp. 1746–1751 (2014)
21. Gao, Y.L., Wu, C., Zhu, M.: Short text classification model based on improved convolutional neural network. J. Jilin Univ. (science edition) **58**(4), 923–930 (2020)
22. Song, J., Zhang, J., Gao, Y.: Comparison of natural language processing and effectiveness of unstructured reporting content of nursing adverse events. J. Nurs. **25**(3), 1–4 (2018)
23. Yin, W., Kann, K., Yu, M., Schütze, H.: Comparative study of CNN and RNN for natural language processing: arXiv preprint arXiv:1702.01923(2017)
24. Bahdanau, D., Cho, K., Bengio, Y.: Neural machine translation by jointly learning to align and translate. Computer Science arXiv:1409.0473 (2014)
25. Li, H., Zheng, Y., Ren, P.: Dual-channel attention model for text sentiment analysis. Int. J. Perform. Eng. **15**(3), 834–841 (2019)
26. Cheng, M., Zhao, X., Ding, X., Gao, J., Xiong, S., Ren, Y.: Prediction of blood culture outcome using hybrid neural network model based on electronic health records. BMC Med. Inform. Decis. Mak. **20**(3), 1–10 (2020)
27. Devlin, J., Chang, M.W., Lee, K., Toutanova, K.: BERT: pre-training of deep bidirectional transformers for language understanding. arXiv preprint arXiv:1810.04805 (2018)
28. Li, X., Zhang, H., Zhou, X.H.: Chinese clinical named entity recognition with variant neural structures based on BERT methods. J. Biomed. Inform. **107**(5), 103422 (2020)
29. Yilmaz, S., Toklu, S.: A deep learning analysis on question classification task using Word2vec representations. Neural Comput. Appl. **32**(7), 2909–2928 (2020). https://doi.org/10.1007/s00521-020-04725-w
30. Dai, B., Li, J., Xu, R.: Multiple positional self-attention network for text classification. In: Proceedings of the AAAI Conference on Artificial Intelligence, vol. 34, pp. 7610–7617 (2020)
31. The Chinese Hospital Association: Quality and safety management of Chinese hospital - Part 4–6: Medical management - Medical safety adverse event management. Standards (2018)

Node Research on the Involvement of China's Carbon Tax Policy in the Context of COVID-19

Huiwen Wu[1], Kanghui Zhang[2,6], Fan Wang[2], Jianhua Liu[7], Wang Zhao[2,3](✉),
Haiqing Xu[1](✉), and Long Lu[2,3,4,5](✉)

[1] Department of Child Health, Maternal and Child Health Hospital of Hubei Province, Wuhan,
China
xuhaiqing9@126.com
[2] School of Information Management, Wuhan University, Wuhan, China
2021101040028@whu.edu.cn, 199223263@qq.com, bioinfo@gmail.com
[3] The Center for Healthcare Big Data Research, The Big Data Institute, Wuhan University,
Wuhan, China
[4] Institute of Pediatrics, Guangzhou Women and Children's Medical Center, Guangzhou
Medical University, Guangzhou, China
[5] School of Public Health, Wuhan University, Wuhan, China
[6] Suzhou Zealikon Healthcare Co., Ltd., Suzhou, China
[7] Child Health Department of Huangshi Maternal and Child Health Hospital, Huangshi, China

Abstract. The outbreak of COVID-19 provides a rare opportunity for the implementation of the carbon tax. To determine which stage is the most appropriate for introducing the policy, a simulation model based on China's panel data is established to analyze the impact of the carbon tax on government revenue and residents' income from five scenarios. A new GM-SD modeling method is proposed to ensure the accuracy of the model. The results show that the impact of the carbon tax on the government and the public is significantly different at different stages, and even the implementation of the carbon tax in the early stage of COVID-19 will reduce the government's tax revenue. The score analysis of government tax revenue, residents' surplus disposable income, residents' emotional value, and government administrative power finds that the middle period of COVID-19 is the best time to implement the policy. In addition, a more detailed analysis of five aspects, including total population, energy consumption, and national income, shows that the best time to implement the carbon tax policy is when the damage degree of COVID-19 is moderate. The analysis results can provide a reference and basis for China to introduce the carbon tax in the event of similar events as COVID-19, and have reference significance for other countries that have not implemented a carbon tax.

Keywords: Carbon tax · GM-SD · COVID-19 · Time node

1 Introduction

In late December 2019, COVID-19 broke out in Wuhan, China. The spread of the epidemic has limited the short-term movement of people, energy demand, and industrial

B. Tang et al. (Eds.): CHIP 2022, CCIS 1772, pp. 197–210, 2023.
https://doi.org/10.1007/978-981-19-9865-2_14

production [1, 2], which had a significant and negative impact on global trade [3], energy prices [4], population size [5], etc. Fernandes' research showed that most countries have seen a drop in GDP of 3–6% as a result of the pandemic, while service-oriented countries have seen a drop of 15.5% [6]. In addition, COVID-19 has caused fluctuations in international oil prices [7]. In 2020, the collapse of the OPEC+ meeting and the epidemic led to a short-term collapse in oil prices [4]. The decline in energy prices has created a valuable opportunity for the introduction of policies to reduce carbon emissions [8].

As an environmental tax, the carbon tax mainly aims at reducing greenhouse gas emissions [9]. It applies to most countries or regions [10]. The main function of the carbon tax is to raise the energy price and reduce the consumption of non-renewable energy [11], so as to achieve emission reduction effect. The outbreak of COVID-19 has unexpectedly achieved the effect of a carbon tax equal to, or even beyond. During the pandemic, global carbon emissions have declined significantly [12]. In early April 2020 alone, global daily CO_2 emissions were 17% lower than the 2019 average, and for the full year, global carbon emissions were 7% lower [2]. This seems to suggest that greenhouse gas emissions can be reduced without policies to reduce emissions. However, it should be noted that the emission reduction effect of the epidemic is short-term and can be ignored [13]. Therefore, new emission reduction policies should be introduced during the pandemic to maintain the level of emission reduction during the pandemic and ensure the sustainability of emission reduction.

Another perceived function of introducing a carbon tax during the pandemic is to stabilize uncontrollable economic fluctuations caused by COVID-19. The outbreak of COVID-19 has reduced the energy demand and caused the price to plummet [14]. In the United States, for example, fuel demand fell sharply during the pandemic, and oil futures prices fell into negative territory in April 2020. In May of the same year, Spanish wholesale electricity prices were 60% lower than expected and gas prices 62% lower than expected [15]. Despite the sharp decline in oil demand, supply remained at pre-pandemic levels, resulting in an oil glut and the full operation of oil storage facilities in some countries for the first time in history [16]. Therefore, introducing a carbon tax is an effective means of raising energy prices, which have fallen due to government lockdown. The involvement of the carbon tax will increase the cost of energy enterprises. To reduce economic risks, energy manufacturers will transfer the cost risks brought by a carbon tax to consumers [17], thus raising energy prices and reducing the drop in energy prices caused by the epidemic.

In addition to maintaining the emission reduction benefits of COVID-19 and stabilizing the market economic fluctuations caused by COVID-19, the carbon tax has another welfare effect, that is, the reinvestment of the tax income can reduce the distorting effects of the existing tax system on capital and labor and improve social welfare [18]. Therefore, compared with the double dividend of the carbon tax [19], the implementation of the carbon tax during the period of COVID-19 will bring an extra dividend, resulting in a triple dividend: emission reduction, social welfare improvement, and market economy stability.

Some scholars have studied the relationship between the epidemic and carbon tax, and all believe that the outbreak period of the epidemic is the perfect time to introduce a carbon tax policy [2, 14, 20]. They argue that introducing a carbon tax in the post-pandemic era would reduce carbon dioxide emissions by increasing investment in alternative renewable energy and reducing the use of non-renewable energy sources. At the same time, the development of renewable energy can create new job opportunities [20], thus reducing the rise in unemployment caused by the epidemic.

The above analysis shows that implementing a carbon tax during the COVID-19 pandemic can amplify the advantages of the policy and reduce the side effects of tax collection. Le Quéré et al. [2] believe that the post-epidemic period was the best time to implement carbon tax policy, but they did not specify the time of introduction. Therefore, from the economic dimension, the paper takes government tax revenue and residents' disposable income as the fulcrum to explore the best time to implement a carbon tax in China under the background of COVID-19 and discusses the impact of implementing carbon tax at the best node under the background of COVID-19 on reducing energy consumption and improving residents' quality of life in two scenarios: COVID-19 and normal.

2 Method

2.1 System Dynamics

System Dynamics (SD) was proposed by Professor Forrester in 1956 [22]. In the beginning, this method is put forward to analyze production management, inventory management, and other enterprise problems. With continuous development, it has gradually become a quantitative research method for complex social and economic systems based on computer simulation technology and feedback control theory [23]. Up to now, SD has become a discipline of analyzing and studying information feedback, and it is also a cross-comprehensive discipline of understanding and solving system problems. SD believes that as long as there is a system, there must be a structure, and the system structure determines the function of the system. According to the feedback characteristics of the internal components of the system, the root cause of the occurrence of problems can be found from the internal structure of the system, rather than using external interference or random events to explain the behavior nature of the system. SD can change from static single-factor real-time analysis to dynamic whole-system analysis [24]. At present, SD has been widely used in the construction industry [25, 26], transportation industry [27], agriculture [28, 29], and so on. The SD modeling and analysis process is detailed in Sects. 2.3 and 3.

2.2 Grey Model

Grey Model (GM) was first proposed by Professor Deng Julong in 1982. With continuous development, it has evolved into the current grey system theory. It is a fusion of information theory, synergetic theory, system theory, structure theory, and mutation theory [30]. GM takes the gray part of the real system as the research object, takes the whitening, desalting, quantization, modeling, and optimization of the gray part of the system as the core, and aims to predict and control the development of the gray part, to achieve the correct description and effective monitoring of the evolution law of the system operation behavior. The prediction principle of GM is to form a group of new data series by using the definite data series with the obvious trend. Secondly, a prediction model is established based on the growing trend of new data series. Finally, the original sequence is restored by subtraction reverse calculation and the prediction results are obtained [31]. The classic grey prediction model is the even GM(1,1) (EGM), which is more widely used than other models. Therefore, the EGM is used to model residents' living expenses in eight aspects, and the established mathematical model is introduced into the system dynamics model of the carbon tax policy.

2.3 GM-SD Modeling

EGM focuses more on the prediction of a single variate. Although some scholars have proposed GM(n, h) model [32] that can achieve multi-variable prediction, it fails to reflect comprehensive systemic changes and the causes of variable changes, thus lacking systematic thinking. The EGM is a prediction method for bleaching, dilution, quantification, modeling, and optimization of a single research object. It focuses more on the data characteristics of the research object itself and ignores the driving effect of other factors on the research object, so it is unable to quantitatively explore the internal mechanism of the change of other factors on the research object. SD model can better compensate for this deficiency. Due to the large number of variables involved in the SD model, the accuracy of the model gradually decreases in the layer-by-layer offset, thus reducing the reliability of the prediction. The grey model can effectively improve the accuracy of the SD model. Therefore, the combination of the two can achieve accurate analysis and prediction of the timing of carbon tax policy intervention, to discover the internal correlation. The combination of the two can achieve accurate analysis and prediction of the timing of the carbon tax policy intervention, to discover the correlation of internal variables.

Figure 1 (left) shows the GM-SD modeling steps. Firstly, it is necessary to clarify the research problem, determine the system boundary, and establish the qualitative causal loop feedback model. Secondly, the necessary data are collected according to the feedback model, the data are preprocessed, and the time-responded function of the sequence was obtained by using EGM. Thirdly, the processed data and time-responded function are imported into the SD model to build the SD simulation model. Fourthly, model checking and testing methods are used to conduct reality checking and numerical trend analysis on the simulation model to ensure the accuracy and robustness of the model. Finally, the simulation model is used to analyze the reality, explore the root of the problem, and then put forward feasible policy suggestions.

The system simulation model (right side of Fig. 1) is established according to the GM-SD modeling steps. First, clarify the question: when is the best time to implement a carbon tax in the context of COVID-19? The strongest correlation with the double dividend of the carbon tax policy is residents' income and government tax revenue respectively, thus conducting causal analysis and variable selection. Second, panel data are collected according to variable selection results and mathematical equations between variables are established. Thirdly, the data and equations are imported into the model to establish the simulation model. Fourthly, the model is validated using mean error and extreme condition test. Fifthly, simulation analysis is conducted to explore the advantages and disadvantages of implementing a carbon tax at different time points and find out the root causes and solutions.

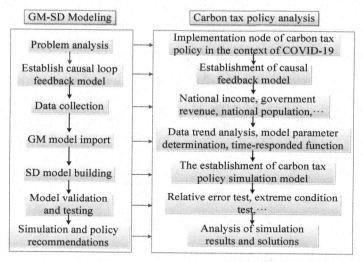

Fig. 1. GM-SD and carbon tax policy modeling steps diagram

3   Establishment and Testing of the Carbon Tax Model

3.1   Establishment of Causal Feedback Model

Figure 2 is the causal feedback model of the carbon tax. The figure shows the causal relationship between variables in the form of arrows. The positive and negative signs of arrows indicate that the relationship between two variables is promoted or inhibited. First of all, government tax revenue directly affects the ability of government departments to deal with emergencies. The spread and severity of the epidemic depend on the government's policies and implementation capacity on the one hand, and the public's trust in the government on the other. The severity of the epidemic will directly affect the public's life, leading to a significant rise or decline in living expenses in many aspects, while the change of living expenses structure will lead to fluctuations in residual disposable income per capita, thus affecting the public's trust in government policies. Therefore, a cause-and-effect cycle model with government tax revenue as the external guide and residents' disposable income as the internal pillar is established.

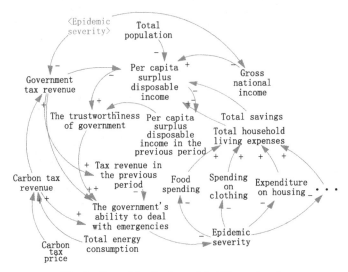

Fig. 2. Causal feedback model of the carbon tax

3.2 Data Sources and Processing

It is necessary to analyze and process the acquired data to reduce the subjectivity of the model and ensure the accuracy of the model. The circular prediction method proposed by Jia and Yan [33] was used to establish the table function of the growth rate in the model. The GM-SD method was used to establish the mathematical formula for the expenditure data of residents. The living expenditure of residents from 2013 to 2019 shows a monotonically increasing sequence with a relatively close growth rate. The government's ability to deal with emergencies and the trustworthiness of the government depend on the comparison between the current period and the previous period, and the delay function is used to realize the comparison relationship. The outbreak of COVID-19 has a fixed point in time. Therefore, the government tax revenue, national income, total population, and other variables are expressed by logical functions. The carbon tax price was set as a fixed value, 50 CNY/ton [18], and represented by a logical function.

3.3 Establishment of Carbon Tax Model

The causal feedback model and the processing results of relevant data provide the core architecture and kernel for the simulation model, respectively. The representation form of the carbon tax model is shown in Fig. 3. Figure 3 specifically divides the variables in Fig. 2. Where, " ☐ " represents the state variable, " ⊠ " represents the rate variable, and others are auxiliary variables.

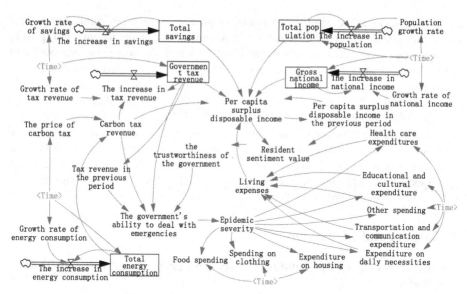

Fig. 3. Simulation model of carbon tax policy

3.4 Model Testing

The robustness of the model is tested by an extreme condition test. SD pays special attention to the influence of parameter variation on system behavior mode [34]. Here, the implementation time of the carbon tax is set as the initial year, and the carbon tax price is set at 0, 10 and 100 respectively, so as to test whether abnormal changes occur in the behavior of the system. A carbon tax directly affects the government's tax revenue, and residual disposable income per capita is the core variable of the model. Choosing these two variables to explain the robustness of the model is more credible, and the simulation results are shown in Fig. 4.

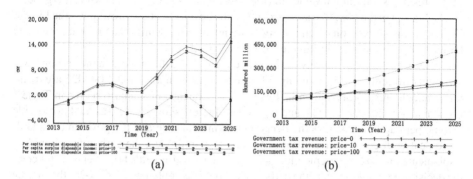

Fig. 4. Extreme condition test

In Fig. 4, (a) is the change of residual disposable income per capita under three carbon tax prices, and (b) is the change of government tax annual income. In Fig. 4(a), when the carbon tax price is 100, the residual disposable income per capita oscillates near 0. This indicates that the income of residents at this time can only meet the needs of basic living and security. At the same time, it also indicates that if China implements the carbon tax before 2025, the carbon tax price should be lower than 100, which confirms the reasonable research results of Zhou et al. [18]. When the carbon tax price is 0, the annual tax revenue is the minimum. With the increase of the carbon tax price, the annual tax revenue of the government increases gradually. When the carbon tax price is 100, the annual tax revenue of the government does not show an unexpected increase or decrease. Under extreme conditions, the key variables of the model do not change significantly, so the model is considered to be robust.

4   Results and Discussion

4.1   Differences in Implementation Effects of a Carbon Tax at Different Time Nodes

When the total amount of social funds remains unchanged, Residual disposable income per capita and government tax revenue are mutually exclusive variables, so how to achieve the balance between them becomes particularly important. Figure 5 shows the simulation results of the influence of implementing the carbon tax on residents and the government at different time nodes. In Fig. 5(a)–(d), normal represents the curve of the normal scenario (no carbon tax is implemented), and tax-2020, tax-2021, and tax-2022 are simulation curves of implementing carbon tax policy in 2020, 2021, and 2022, respectively.

Figure 5 shows that under different evaluation dimensions, levying carbon tax at different periods has advantages and disadvantages. Taking the simulation value at 2021 as an example, the values of four variables in the tax-2020 scenario are all the lowest compared with the other three scenarios. In 2022, the residual disposable income per capita, residents' emotional value, and the government's ability to deal with emergencies are the highest in the tax-2020 scenario, while the government's tax revenue is the lowest. Therefore, the simulation results in Fig. 5 are not able to identify the optimal time point for carbon tax collection during the COVID-19 pandemic.

In order to comprehensively evaluate and identify the differences in the carbon taxes levied in different periods, four variables under four scenarios in 2020–2025 are quantified, and the results are shown in Table 1. The sequence of scenario scores in Table 1 is (normal, tax-2020, tax-2021, and tax-2022). Table 1 shows that if residual disposable income per capita is taken as the decision-making variable and the government's ability to deal with emergencies during COVID-19 is improved, the carbon tax should be implemented in 2020 (pre-epidemic period). If the government's tax revenue is taken as the decision-making variable, the carbon tax should be implemented in 2021 (the middle of the pandemic). If resident sentiment value is taken as the decision-making variable, the carbon tax should not be implemented during the COVID-19 period. When taking benefit maximization as the standard, Table 1 does not show that implementing a carbon tax in the post-COVID-19 period is the optimal choice. However, in Table 1, the scores

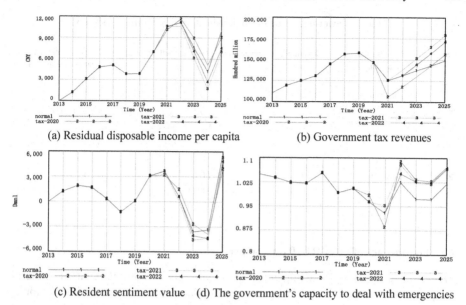

(a) Residual disposable income per capita   (b) Government tax revenues

(c) Resident sentiment value   (d) The government's capacity to deal with emergencies

Fig. 5. Assessment of variables under different scenarios

of tax-2022 scenarios are all higher than 2, and one value is less than 2 in the other three scenarios, which may be the reason why many scholars believe that carbon tax policy is implemented in the post-epidemic period. A comprehensive weighted analysis was performed on the mean values in Table 1. The scoring results are ((9.83), (9.99), (10.16), (9.99)). This overall score shows that the tax-2021 scenario is optimal, i.e. the introduction of a carbon tax in the middle of the COVID-19 pandemic.

In Fig. 5, a paradox against cognition appears: after the implementation of the carbon tax in 2020, residents' surplus disposable income will be higher in 2022–2024 than that without a carbon tax, while government tax revenue is on the contrary. The reason behind this phenomenon is that price of commodities has been maintained due to the carbon tax imposed by the government in 2020, and households have further cut back on consumption due to the COVID-19 pandemic, which has led to an increase in residents' disposable income and a decrease in government tax revenue. In addition, in the model, residents' emotions and the government's ability to deal with emergencies are not determined by the total income of the residents and government, but by the remaining income of the residents and government tax revenue in the previous period. This leads to the high emotional value of residents in the tax-2020 scenario in 2022 and 2023, and the government has the highest ability to deal with emergencies after 2022.

Table 1. Quantified value of implementation time of the carbon tax

Year	Residual disposable income per capita	Government tax revenues	Resident sentiment value	The government's capacity to deal with emergencies
2020	(2.5),(2.5),(2.5),(2.5)	(2.5),(2.5),(2.5),(2.5)	(2.5),(2.5),(2.5),(2.5)	(2),(4),(2),(2)
2021	(3),(1),(3),(3)	(3),(1),(3),(3)	(3),(1),(3),(3)	(2.5),(1),(4),(2.5)
2022	(2.5),(4),(1),(2.5)	(2.5),(1),(4),(2.5)	(2.5),(1),(4),(2.5)	(1),(4),(3),(2)
2023	(3),(4),(1),(2)	(2),(1),(4),(3)	(3),(4),(1),(2)	(1),(4),(2),(3)
2024	(3),(4),(1),(2)	(1.5),(1.5),(4),(3)	(4),(3),(1.5),(1.5)	(1),(4),(2),(3)
2025	(4),(3),(1),(2)	(2),(1),(4),(3)	(4),(1),(3),(2)	(1),(4),(2),(3)
mean value	(3),(3.08),(1.58),(2.33)	(2.25),(1.33),(3.58),(2.83)	(3.16),(2.08),(2.5),(2.25)	(1.42),(3.5),(2.5),(2.58)

4.2 The Impact of COVID-19 on Society

To further analyze the optimal implementation time of the carbon tax, economics, energy, and population induced by COVID-19 were simulated and compared with the normal scenario. The results are shown in Fig. 6. As can be seen from Fig. 6, government tax revenue is the factor most severely affected by the epidemic (Fig. 6(c)), which has a smaller impact on China's population than other variables (Fig. 6(b)). The research results of Wang et al. [5] also showed that the number of deaths caused by COVID-19 in China was less than that in other countries. The lockdown policy of the Chinese government has resulted in a severe impact on enterprise production, which in turn has an impact on national income and energy consumption (Fig. 6(a) and (d)). Residents' living expenses were mainly affected by the blockade policy. When the blockade policy was almost lifted, residents' living expenses returned to normal (Fig. 6(e)).

For China, the implementation of a carbon tax should consider the changes in government revenue, national income, and energy consumption, and at the same time, we should be aware of the paradox caused by the implementation of the carbon tax. Figure 6 shows that compared with other variables, COVID-19 has a greater impact on China's government tax revenue, but the early stage of COVID-19 is not the best time to impose a carbon tax to restore the government's administrative power. Figure 5(b) shows that the implementation of the carbon tax in the early stage of COVID-19 will result in lower government revenue than that without the implementation of the carbon tax. Implementing a carbon tax in the early stages of COVID-19 may produce a more effective reduction, i.e. lower energy consumption than in Fig. 6(d) in the COVID-19 scenario. But such misshapen emission reduction could provoke a popular backlash. Implementing a carbon tax in the mid-pandemic has a predictable positive effect on revenue and emission reduction. Firstly, in the mid-pandemic, social productivity and labor force are in a semi-liberated state. The intervention of the carbon tax will restrain the surge in social material demand and imbalance between supply and demand caused by the lifting of the lockdown policy, and provide a positive micro-stimulus to the sustainable development of society, thus continuing the advantages of COVID-19 in reducing emissions. Secondly, based on reasonably reducing material demand, the emergence of a carbon tax will increase tax revenue and enhance the government's ability to regulate the social system. The secondary distribution of carbon tax revenue can effectively help the audiences most affected by COVID-19. Finally, the distorting effects of a carbon tax on households' living expenses will be weakened and reduced during the COVID-19 pandemic. Therefore, implementing the carbon tax policy in the mid-pandemic has objective positive benefits.

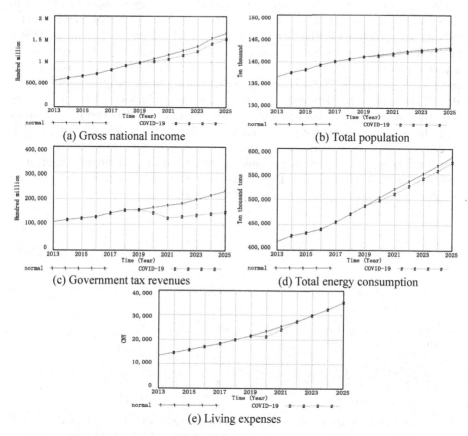

(a) Gross national income

(b) Total population

(c) Government tax revenues

(d) Total energy consumption

(e) Living expenses

Fig. 6. Comparison between normal scenario and COVID-19 scenario

4.3   Carbon Tax and Residents' Expenditure

Figure 7 shows the simulation and comparison results of residents' expenditure in various aspects of life under normal scenarios and the COVID-19 scenario in 2020 and 2021. From the comparison of the histogram of figures (a) and (b), it can be seen that the living expenditure of residents increases gradually over time, and the living expenditure of residents is affected by the severity of COVID-19. This suggests that COVID-19 can reduce energy consumption for the population as a whole. The implementation of a carbon tax can replace COVID-19 to maintain the level of household spending, reduce market fluctuations caused by the epidemic, and stabilize social order. Compared to the normal scenario, COVID-19 will lead to a 10–15% decrease in living expenses in 2020 and a 5–8% decrease in 2021. Therefore, the carbon tax in the early stage of COVID-19 can maintain such a low energy consumption state, which can maximize energy consumption savings, but this decrease is at the cost of completely curbing household expenditure. The implementation of a carbon tax policy in the mid-term of COVID-19 can not only stabilize the social and economic market but also restrain excessive energy consumption of residents and improve the effectiveness of energy conservation and emission reduction. Implementing a carbon tax in the post-pandemic is less effective in reducing emissions than in the middle part of the pandemic.

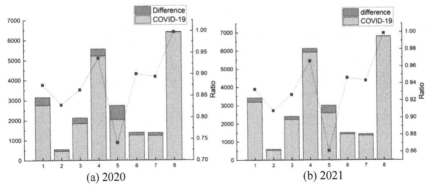

Fig. 7. Comparison of expenditure on all aspects of living under normal scenario and COVID-19 scenario. (1. Transportation and communication expenditure; 2. Other spending; 3. Health care expenditures; 4. Expenditure on housing; 5. Educational and cultural expenditure. 6. Expenditure on daily necessities; 7. Spending on clothing; 8. Food spending)

Figure 7 shows that the change ratio of residents' food expenditure is the smallest, and education and culture expenditure is the largest. According to the expenditure of residents in all aspects of life under the COVID-19 scenario, the expenditure on education and culture, other expenditures, and medical care can be properly controlled and reduced, while the expenditure on food, housing, daily necessities, and clothing should not be suppressed. Therefore, the carbon tax should be implemented after the basic recovery of household essential expenditure. Figure 7(b) shows that residents' food consumption expenditure in 2021 is infinitely close to 1, which indicates that implementing a carbon tax in the mid-term of COVID-19 can effectively reduce non-renewable energy consumption based on guaranteeing residents' life. In the post-epidemic period, residents' basic living expenses are completely stable, coupled with residents' perceptual adaptation response, which may weaken the effectiveness of the carbon tax.

References

1. Bahmanyar, A., Estebsari, A., Ernst, D.: The impact of different COVID-19 containment measures on electricity consumption in Europe. Energy Res. Soc. Sci. **68**, 101683 (2020)
2. Le Quéré, C., et al.: Temporary reduction in daily global CO2 emissions during the COVID-19 forced confinement. Nat. Climate Change **10**(7), 647–653 (2020)
3. Abu-Rayash, A., Dincer, I.: Analysis of mobility trends during the COVID-19 Coronavirus pandemic: exploring the impacts on global aviation and travel in selected cities. Energy Res. Soc. Sci. **68**, 101693 (2020)
4. Jia, Z., Wen, S., Lin, B.: The effects and reacts of COVID-19 pandemic and international oil price on energy, economy, and environment in China. Appl. Energy **302**, 117612 (2021)
5. Wang, H., Paulson, K.P., Pease, S.A., et al.: Estimating excess mortality due to the COVID-19 pandemic: a systematic analysis of COVID-19-related mortality, 2020–21. Lancet **399**(10334), 1513–1536 (2022)
6. Fernandes, N.: Economic effects of coronavirus outbreak (COVID-19) on the world economy. IESE Business School Working Paper No. WP-1240-E (2020)
7. Narayan, P.K.: Oil price news and COVID-19 - is there any connection. Energy Res. Lett. **1**(1), 1–4 (2021)
8. Mintz-Woo, K., Dennig, F., Liu, H., Schinko, T.: Carbon pricing and COVID-19. Climate Policy **21**(10), 1272–1280 (2021)
9. Zhou, Y., Fang, W., Li, M., Liu, W.: Exploring the impacts of a low-carbon policy instrument: a case of carbon tax on transportation in China. Resour. Conserv. Recycl. **139**, 307–314 (2018)
10. Sumner, J., Bird, L., Smith, H.: Carbon taxes: a review of experience and policy design considerations. Climate Policy **11**(2), 922–943 (2009)
11. Yuan, C., Liu, S., Wu, J.: The relationship among energy prices and energy consumption in China. Energy Policy **38**(1), 197–207 (2010)
12. Barbier, E.B., Burgess, J.C.: Sustainability and development after COVID-19. World Dev. **135**, 105082 (2020)
13. Forster, P.M., et al.: Current and future global climate impacts resulting from COVID-19. Nat. Clim. Chang. **10**(10), 913–919 (2020)
14. Zhang, L., Li, H., Lee, W.J., Liao, H.: COVID-19 and energy: influence mechanisms and research methodologies. Sustain. Prod. Consumption **27**(6), 2134–2152 (2021)
15. Abadie, L.M.: Energy market prices in times of covid-19: the case of electricity and natural gas in Spain. Energies **14**(6), 1632 (2021)
16. Bildirici, M., Bayazit, N.G., Ucan, Y.: Analyzing crude oil prices under the impact of COVID-19 by using lstargarchlstm. Energies **13**(11), 1–18 (2020)
17. Khastar, M., Aslani, A., Nejati, M.: How does carbon tax affect social welfare and emission reduction in Finland? Energy Rep. **6**, 736–744 (2020)
18. Coady, D., Parry, I., Sears, L., Shang, B.: How large are global fossil fuel subsidies? World Dev. **91**, 11–27 (2017)
19. Speck, S.: Energy and carbon taxes and their distributional implications. Energy Policy **27**(11), 659–667 (1999)
20. Malliet, P., Reynès, F., Landa, G., Hamdi-Cherif, M., Saussay, A.: Assessing short-term and long-term economic and environmental effects of the COVID-19 crisis in France. Environ. Resource Econ. **76**(4), 867–883 (2020). https://doi.org/10.1007/s10640-020-00488-z

21. Hosseini, S.E.: An outlook on the global development of renewable and sustainable energy at the time of Covid-19. Energy Res. Soc. Sci. **68**, 101633 (2020)

22. Forrester, J.W.: Sustainable Development Strategy of Industry. Scientific American, California (1989)

23. Chen, Z., Zhang, K., Jia, S.: "Green Paradox" effect of new-energy vehicles based on system dynamics. Oper. Res. Manage. Sci. **30**(03), 232–239 (2021). (In Chinese)

24. Hjorth, P., Bagheri, A.: Navigating towards sustainable development: a system dynamics approach. Futures **38**(1), 74–92 (2006)

25. Teng, J., Wang, P., Wu, X., Xu, C.: Decision-making tools for evaluation the impact on the eco-footprint and eco-environmental quality of green building development policy. Sustain. Cities Soc. **23**, 50–58 (2016)

26. Li, Q., Zhang, L., Zhang, L., Jha, S.: Exploring multi-level motivations towards green design practices: a system dynamics approach. Sustain. Cities Soc. **64**, 102490 (2021)

27. Trappey, A.J.C., Trappey, C., Hsiao, C.T., Ou, J.J.R., Li, S.J., Chen, K.W.P.: An evaluation model for low carbon island policy: the case of Taiwan's green transportation policy. Energy Policy **45**, 510–515 (2012)

28. Dace, E., Muizniece, I., Blumberga, A., Kaczalab, F.: Searching for solutions to mitigate greenhouse gas emissions by agricultural policy decisions—application of system dynamics modeling for the case of Latvia. Sci. Total Environ. **527**, 80–90 (2015)

29. Li, F.J., Dong, S.C., Li, F.: A system dynamics model for analyzing the eco-agriculture system with policy recommendations. Ecol. Model. **227**, 34–45 (2012)

30. Li, S.: Grey System Theory and Its Application. Science Press, Beijing (2017). (In Chinese)

31. Wang, Q., Li, S., Zhang, M., Li, R.: Impact of COVID-19 pandemic on oil consumption in the United States: a new estimation approach. Energy **239**, 122280 (2022)

32. Xie, N., Liu, S.: Study on the characteristics of GM(n, h) modeling sequence data multiplicative transformation. Control Decis. **24**(09), 1294–1299 (2009). (In Chinese)

33. Jia, S., Yan, G.: Effects of the policy of air pollution charging fee based on system dynamics and grey model approach. Syst. Eng. Theory Pract. **39**(09), 2436–2450 (2019). (In Chinese)

34. Su, M., Wang, H.: Sensitivity analysis of system dynamics model. Syst. Eng. **04**, 7–12 (1988). (In Chinese)

Author Index

B. Tang et al. (Eds.): CHIP 2022, CCIS 1772, pp. 211–212, 2023.
https://doi.org/10.1007/978-981-19-9865-2

Printed in the United States
by Baker & Taylor Publisher Services